Rowing without Oars

Rowing without Oars

Ulla-Carin Lindquist

Translated by Margaret Myers

VIKING

VIKING

Published by the Penguin Group

Penguin Group (USA) Inc., 375 Hudson Street, New York, New York 10014, U.S.A.
• Penguin Group (Canada), 90 Eglinton Avenue East, Suite 700, Toronto, Ontario,
Canada M4P 2Y3 (a division of Pearson Penguin Canada Inc.) • Penguin Books Ltd,
80 Strand, London WC2R 0RL, England • Penguin Ireland, 25 St. Stephen's Green,
Dublin 2, Ireland (a division of Penguin Books Ltd) • Penguin Books Australia Ltd,
250 Camberwell Road, Camberwell, Victoria 3124, Australia
(a division of Pearson Australia Group Pty Ltd) • Penguin Books India Pvt Ltd,
11 Community Centre, Panchsheel Park, New Delhi – 110 017, India • Penguin Group (NZ),
Cnr Airborne and Rosedale Roads, Albany, Auckland 1310,
New Zealand (a division of Pearson New Zealand Ltd) • Penguin Books
(South Africa) (Pty) Ltd, 24 Sturdee Avenue, Rosebank, Johannesburg 2196, South Africa

Penguin Books Ltd, Registered Offices:
80 Strand, London WC2R 0RL, England

First American edition
Published in 2006 by Viking Penguin,
a member of Penguin Group (USA) Inc.

1 3 5 7 9 10 8 6 4 2

Originally published in Swedish as *Ro utan åror* by Norstedts Forlag, Stockholm.
English-language edition first published in Great Britain by John Murray (Publishers)

Excerpt from "Over the Rainbow" by Harold Arlen and E.Y. Harburg. © 1938 (renewed
1966) Metro-Goldwyn-Mayer Inc. © 1939 (renewed 1967) EMI Feist Catalog Inc. Rights
throughout the world controlled by EMI Feist Catalog Inc. (publishing) and Alfred Publishing
Co., Inc. (print). All rights reserved. Used by permission.

LIBRARY OF CONGRESS CATALOGING IN PUBLICATION DATA

Lindquist, Ulla-Carin, d. 2004.
[Ro utan åror. English]
Rowing without oars / Ulla-Carin Lindquist ; translated by Margaret Myers.
p. cm.
ISBN 0-670-03475-4
1. Lindquist, Ulla-Carin, d. 2004. 2. Amyotrophic lateral sclerosis—Patients—Biography. I. Title.

RC406.A24L56 2006
362.196'839'0092—dc22   2005042437

Printed in the United States of America

To the best of all:
My children Ulrica, Carin, Pontus and Gustaf
And to my beloved Olle

With thanks to Aina Bergvall

Translation in memory of Marie Nebeská, who died of ALS in November 2003, vibrant, courageous and loving to the end.

This is where I begin and where I end.

It is about my end.

Not a memoir as one might imagine such a book.

More like a diary of thoughts and quick flights into my memory, which I have written down. And a number of interviews and factual observations.

'Halfway' through my life I have been invaded by a rare disease, amyotrophic lateral sclerosis, ALS. It has a fast and aggressive course. There is only one end: death. No cure. No recovery.

What happens to a person in this situation?

A year ago I was a full-time TV reporter. Today I cannot eat without help, walk or wash myself.

I feel profound sorrow about everything I am not going to experience. I am devastated that soon I will leave my four children.

At the same time I feel great joy and happiness about everything I am experiencing at the moment. Several times a day my house is filled with laughter.

Does that sound strange?

January 2004

The boat has a heavy motor. It is difficult to put in to the shore in the stiff north-easterly.

'I'll shut off the motor. We'll have to row to the jetty,' shouts Olle, and the head-wind tugs at his rain-jacket. It billows out behind him like a parachute.

'OK,' I yell, and grab the oars. A strong current runs round the point of the island and I stand up to gather my strength.

There is a driving wind and I have to strain with every muscle.

But the oars are as heavy as lead.

As though they were frozen into the water.

Impossible to budge.

Another try.

My hand slides.

There's a sudden burning in my right palm as the oar cuts into it.

I can't row!

'What's the matter with you? You have no strength in your muscles any more.'

Humiliated, angry and near to tears. The usual feeling of inadequacy.

'Row yourself, then, damn it!'

And he does just that.

We load food supplies and wine bottles into the bicycle-cart and struggle up the slope. The boys run on ahead and feed the sheep.

'You've no strength for anything these days, Usse.'

He stares at me, with a new expression.

Now, afterwards, he tells me that at that instant he realised his wife had lost control. That something was wrong.

My Granny's hands, playing. Long, knobbly fingers, with veins like earthworms, deep furrows between the knuckles. Bony and sinewy.

It is these I see in the sunshine when I stretch up with laundered white towels towards the line slung between two pines. The earth of the islands is parched and in the coming days there will be a thunderstorm. Lightning will strike, making the neighbour's plates crash to the floor. Our home will become dark.

But not today. Today the September sun is warm and the Indian summer cradles us in new hope.

I don't know that my nerves are teetering on the brink.

That their life is measured in seconds.

That I have lost my grip.

The clothes-pegs are grey, wind-ravaged. Hauling the sheet over the line is heavy work. My arm moves as usual. It changes gear from first to third by delaying a while in neutral. It is less painful that way. But I can't press open this clothes-peg.

Or any other. I have no strength.

Instead I have a hollow between my thumb and index finger.

A muscle has disappeared and my hand has turned into Granny's. That much is clear.

'Hi, Pontus is ill. They rang from his nursery school. He's throwing up. You'll have to fetch him.'

'Me? I can't. I'm about to operate on a burns case.'

'But I have to be on the air! I have masses to prepare.'

'They're calling me from the operating theatre now. It's a bad case. Bye-bye.' He hangs up.

Everyone around the news desk hears our conversation.

Who is the 'winner'? The plastic surgeon with a person's life in his hands or the newsreader with two million viewers?

'It's not really a choice, is it?' says my editor.

And there are endless queues of newsreaders who long to work on the country's major news programme.

I stop work, travel home and take care of a sick boy.

To be the mother of small children, thus having two jobs, is as exhausting for me as it is for everyone else.

Perhaps with the difference that everyone can see how little sleep I've had.

'Dear me, you did look tired this evening. Are you coping?' wonders Mummy, in Värmland.

The days when I present the main show are long. Get up just after six, wash and blow-dry my hair – it has to look perfect – listen to the morning news, wake the children, make the porridge, log on to the computer, dress small boys, drive to the day nursery, home again, make the beds, walk to the train. Breathe out. Read the morning newspapers' comment columns. If there aren't many, I have time to skim through the culture pages. What luxury!

Twenty-five minutes' brisk walk from the station to the TV building. The morning meeting. On trial. 'What made you evaluate the news that way?' Anxiety in my stomach: will I be criticised? I have always been afraid of that.

News flows in from Indonesia, Moscow, Norrköping, Sundsvall, Washington, Cape Town and Parliament.

Fast tempo, abrupt U-turns.

'No! That won't do. You've got no balls. Rewrite it!' screams the newsroom's Iron Lady, the evening's editor, to a reporter, and swings her crocodile-skin boots up on to the desk.

An outsider would probably be intimidated by our language. But we need it in the buzz of news where torture victims, war-wounded and the homeless are mixed with bribery, economic scandals and Questions to the House.

There is no cheerful news today so I choose a dark blue jacket, a bone-white silk shirt and pearls. Below the waist doesn't matter. It can't be seen.

'I thought you sat on wheels and were rolled into a cupboard after the show,' a man in the street once told me.

If he only knew.

News headlines. News summaries. Everything is written at breakneck speed. Facts are checked. Features shortened, rewritten. Thrown away. Dumped. New information. Rewrite!

Take two steps at a time.

'You must never take the lift up to the studio. What if it got stuck?'

The makeup people are always calm: foundation, powder, blusher, eye-shadow and mascara.

'Is Moscow ready?'

The signature tune and red light. We're on the air.

'Go to the next feature. We've lost Moscow,' whispers the Iron Lady, in my earpiece.

Good evening!

I improvise. A newsreader must be able to do that.

And we can.

It's a passable show. Some viewers ring in with opinions on the feature from the West Bank.

I get home just in time to say goodnight to the boys.

'Mummy, today I kissed you on the TV,' says Gustaf, 'but you didn't kiss me back.'

'I'm doing it now.'

'Night-night.'

'Night-night. Sleep well.'

When we arrived home at Arlanda airport I felt as though I knew every second person. Eleven hours' travelling and the time shift had certainly confused me, but most people looked as though they had sprung from my family in Värmland.

'It's because everyone is fair-haired, of course,' said Olle.

In Montréal in Québec, Canada, genuine blondes are rare. The descendants of the French are often more French than the French; their hair is black and their eyes are dark brown.

Our sons, Olle and I had lived there for two years.

I'm glad about that.

Olle had operated on severe burns patients at one of the city's hospitals and I helped out in the school sick bay. Four children of my own and common sense were all the training I needed.

The first time I got on to a bus on Sherbrooke, the avenue that crosses the city, it struck me that everyone was utterly indifferent to me.

I looked around but nobody took the slightest notice of me. I soon realised that it was because I was just one of the crowd.

I'm slightly ashamed to admit it now, but I was so used to people staring at me when I got on to the bus in Stockholm that it felt strange when they didn't in Montréal.

However.

What freedom. A blank page.

Not once have I regretted leaving my job as a news-reader. Although I loved it.

My GP asks me to strip to the waist. 'You're athletically built.'

He examines my spine. 'Lift your arm sideways. Now forward. And straight up . . . You're exceedingly straight-backed. Like a poker. But your right shoulder isn't as mobile as the left.'

A referral to have an X-ray of my neck and the cervical part of my spine. Magnetic Resonance Imaging (MRI). Without comment. It reveals a minor slipped disc. An incidental discovery. Probably irrelevant in this context.

Contact my good friend who is a professor of neuro-physiology. Why not before now? Ulnaris, medianus and radialis. The nerves of the hand have names that sound like Swedish adoptive surnames. Brachialis. Dorsalis. A new world opens up and I am fascinated by synapses, axons and nerve endings. All in finely tuned harmony.

A balance between nerves and muscles. Like the perfection and sonority of a well-rehearsed symphony orchestra.

But here something is out of tune.

What?

I return to the newsroom, but not as a newsreader. I've finished with that. The years in Canada have freed me from the yoke of needing to be seen on television, which was once my *raison d'être*. I am now going to look after consumer affairs.

I am happy and free, and I fly down the stairs at Östra station. I'm wearing my new Armani jeans and take three steps at a time.

A forty-nine-year-young woman reconquers the world.

Consumer affairs need to be given more time in the news. I email and ring consumer advisers, lawyers, eco-police and market economists to build a network of contacts. I fly to Gothenburg on a research trip and the resulting feature is headlined in the news broadcasts.

The only thing I miss is a nimble right hand for taking notes.

One visit to the doctor is followed by another.

'Up to now we've had invitations to dinner and parties on the fridge. Now there are only your summonses to the doctor,' jokes Olle.

Neurophysiologist Sture Hansson's hands are warm as he touches my body. Carefully, he inserts electrodes, the size of acupuncture needles. He is interested in his work and I, too, become fascinated by what he sees on the computer screen, the muscles' electrical activity, and I forget that it hurts a little. When it bleeds he puts on a plaster.

'On one occasion a patient rang me after I'd examined him and told me he'd recovered. The electrode needles had worked like acupuncture for him,' Dr Hansson tells me.

But for me today's examination is depressing. The nerves in my right arm and hand are measurably damaged: it is possible to see twitchings right up to my shoulder. When I nag stubbornly for information Dr Hansson refers me to the neurologist.

'Have you ever been badly injured?' asks the woman who has become my neurologist. Her name is Anne Zachau and she is a cross between Snow White and a ballerina. I feel profound respect for her.

Certainly, I have galloped in wild terrain. I have crashed straight into a fence when a horse bolted. I've tumbled all the way down a black ski run. Shortened sail in a gale and was knocked on the head by the boom. Had to brake suddenly, then fell on long-distance skates. I put a stop to judo when the throws became too rough for a mother of small children.

'Did you ever have to go to hospital?'

'No,' I reply, but I tell her that my mother had to cancel two patients once when I was five and became king of the castle over my eight-year-old brother. I got to the top of a pile of frozen leaves first. He was angry and bashed my head with a broken stool. I ran to the surgery and sat down on a waiting-room chair and waited for Mummy to finish drilling a tooth. In the end I raised my voice a little and said, 'Mummy, it's raining outside. I'm wet.'

It was a crystal clear, sunny October day. She turned and saw her daughter with blood running down her face. The hospital stitched me, and the smell of ether would remind me for ever of hospitals.

Dr Zachau smiles a little and asks me to put out my tongue. She studies it carefully looking for nerve twitches, fasciculations. She sees none. That is good. It indicates that the nerve damage is peripheral, in the lower motor neurone, which is not in the brain. Those injuries do not heal.

I am ashamed of the yellowish coating on my tongue and thankful to be allowed to shut my mouth.

The journalist in me searches the web. I fear the worst. Most things can be found on the web and I become obsessed with the search for more. Motor-neurone disease. MS. Bulbar pares. Amyotrophic lateral sclerosis.

ALS?

There can be too much information. Short-circuit in my confused brain.

I let myself be enticed by the minor slipped disc that the MRI revealed. Of all the doctors I have consulted, only one has said that a slipped disc can give rise to symptoms like mine. It sounds safe, and is something on which it is possible to use a knife.

My friend Johan accompanies me to the Stockholm Spine Centre at Löwenströmska Hospital. The autumn weather is wet and windy and the window on the driver's side of my Peugeot suddenly drops with a bang. The wind blows in, we hang a blanket over the gap and laugh.

The doctor, a well-known neurosurgeon, is late. He receives me half reclining in his chair.

He's a sailor, I think, as he asks me to take off everything except my panties and bra. No screen or curtain. A chair to put my trousers and jacket on.

Black panties and bra have seldom felt so out of place. I lower my eyes self-consciously and discover that I am standing on a Persian carpet.

'Stretch out your arm.

'Lift your left leg.

'Turn your head sideways.'

I pin my eyes on Marilyn Monroe's lips in black-and-white. The picture is neatly framed and stands on the bookshelf in the room where the doctor examines his patients.

I stand in black underwear with my arm outstretched on the dark red carpet and stare at Marilyn Monroe.

It is not because of the slipped disc that my hand is paralysed. The slipped disc is on the wrong side for that.

When Johan and I take the E18 motorway home, the wind blows harder through the hole where the car window recently was.

More examinations. More needles and electric impulses measure the deterioration of my muscles and nerves.

The spinal-fluid test makes me feel as though I were wrapped in a temporary shroud. I am anchored in the depths of the sea for six days.

When I have surfaced again, a couple of kilos lighter, I buy a button-buttoner, a tin-opener, some tongs, an angled knife, a pen and scissors in the handicap shop.

I am an astronaut. A helmet is pushed on to my head. A control panel for communication. A mirror to see out. Then, slowly, into the monster.

I am in a coffin. A crematorium. The fire flares up.

'No, an astronaut! Not a damned corpse!' Panic.

Knock, knock, knock, knock, knock, a hundred knock-knockings, and twice as many drone-dronings.

Soon I shall know everything about MRIs. Seven times into the tunnel. Even the tiniest pocket in the labyrinth of my brain has been ransacked.

It takes time to unpack the removal crates with my feeble right hand. There are also the dozens of boxes that remained in the cellar during our two years in Canada.

I fumble and drop things.

It's quite normal nowadays.

Probably has something to do with age and that I'm always in a hurry to get things done.

Luckily I have plenty of stamina, thanks to having jogged and walked round almost the whole of Montréal. I got to know the town in a pair of Nikes . . .

A bagel, the risen dough dipped in boiling water laced with honey, then baked in a wood-fired oven, with smoked salmon, Philadelphia cream cheese and capers, is what I bought on the Rue St Viateur and ate up on Mont Royal.

From the top of the hill, 223 metres high, you can see as far as the much higher peaks in Vermont, USA.

The countryside around my newly conquered city is flat.

The boys are Scouts, and when I sew beaver badges on to their blue shirts I complain about the shoddiness of Canadian needles. My seams are clumsy and ugly.

And that can't be my fault.

Pens are of poor quality too. I get cramps in my hands when I write.

The skin on the potatoes is too thick or the potato-peeler is no good.

The list continues.

On my forty-eighth and forty-ninth birthdays – as on every birthday, now I'm middle-aged – I do backbends and stand on my head, without support, with my legs at an angle of ninety degrees, to check my physical fitness and co-ordination.

But now, here at home in Sweden, my strength is ebbing.

Perhaps it's the change that's making me tired?

Complaints about pain are so tedious, but my shoulders feel as though they are strung up on a girder.

And the boxes are so heavy.

I keep tripping.

Surely the lawn wasn't always so uneven?

The autumn of 2002 consists simply of endless assessments and treatments by different physiotherapists. Somebody shakes her head and says there is nothing she can do.

The winter passes in half-darkness. I fall prey to feeling sorry for myself when I am unable to wrap the Christmas presents. I can't even contemplate tying a bow – way back in the autumn I couldn't tie my shoelaces – or writing gift-tags.

The spectre inside me whispers, 'Perhaps this is your last Christmas.'

I hate self-pity. But for a while that's where I end up.

'We'll wait and see what happens.'

The physiotherapists take over from each other. Someone straps up my shoulder, someone applies a wet, warm compress to my stomach, and someone else gives me a workout.

One day my right leg bends backwards when I am on a brisk winter walk.

A warning bell.

Another day the nerve twitchings begin in my left arm, like tiny bubbles: the first kicks of a foetus.

Now I am off sick part-time and have free medical treatment. But I can still go on the family skiing holiday to Switzerland where Olle's sister lives.

I manage to ski and get down quite tough slopes with only one stick.

One day we pass a nameplate:

'Dr med. Christoph v. Hippel, Facharzt FMH für Neurologie'.

On the spot I am given an appointment for the following day.

And he is convinced that I have a motor-neurone disease, not an injury.

The word for patience in Arabic is 'cactus'. They have the same meaning – 'to endure thirst'.

I buy a cactus and ponder. It's as the poet Karin Boye wrote, the best day is a day of thirst.

Surely I shall be able to endure adversity and have the courage to steel myself?

The Nobel Prize winner Imre Kertész helps too. The teenage boy in *Man Without a Past* adapts and survives. He takes what happens in Auschwitz as a matter of course. He adapts.

I decide to do that too.

Observe. Adapt.

Step by step.

My right hand droops more with each day that passes. At the same time, the fingers become stiffer, more bent. In the morning when I wake up my hand is locked, clenched.

'You ought to have a cradle-splint,' says the newsroom's young medical reporter. She also has problems with a hand and we often complain to each other.

People react in different ways. 'Oh, well . . . you still have your left hand,' says the one who believes in positive thinking.

'Now you know what it's like to get old before your time,' says the person who is bitter.

'Think about all those who lose a hand working a machine,' says the labour reporter.

But when somebody bursts out, 'How awful! It's blue – just look at it!' it is I who says, 'Oh, well, it's not that bad. I still have my left hand.'

The medical reporter persuades me to go to the district occupational therapist. She is to be found at a nursing home for the elderly.

'Is it ALS, do you think?' I ask while she warms a piece of plastic in an electric wok.

I have one like it at home for making Thai food.

The therapist cuts the softened plastic, and tries to mould it to my arm, but the arm is so stiff that this is impossible. I have to lie down. The county council needs to save money so she cuts the Velcro lengthwise. She is deft with her fingers – but then, she does embroidery in her spare time.

'If it's ALS . . . I'm no doctor . . . You're surely too young for that.'

She tells me that she has met eight or ten ALS patients during the past ten years. All older than I am.

'You've probably got a peripheral injury in the outer nerve circuit. It should heal. But, as I said, I'm no doctor.'

Hope she's right.

I feel satisfied when I drive away from there. So does my hand, as it lies in its cradle.

Friday 4 April is hectic. When the shops open I buy a new top for the party this evening. At twelve o'clock I'm due in Neurophysiology at Uppsala University Hospital for an examination. We have to allow an hour for the journey. My neighbour will drive me.

I try to jot down a few notes for the speech I have to give this evening.

Thirty guests have been invited.

About the right number, I think.

Seated dinner.

Fun.

At Uppsala there is equipment they still don't have at Karolinska Hospital. It measures the functioning of the nerves from the brain and can determine whether or not the twitches and paralysis in my hand are due to an injury to the central nervous system.

I like the doctor, who has just arrived home from a golf trip to Turkey. He is concerned.

My right hand doesn't register on the machine. My left arm and leg are normal: 'No comment'.

My right leg lies motionless. No reaction.

No signal.

Nothing.

'What does it mean?' I ask, although I already know the answer.

It is quiet in the room.

'It's not my business to give you an answer,' replies the neurophysiologist, hesitantly. 'Your neurologist should tell you.'

'But I'm sure it's ALS.'

'Do you really want to know?'

'Perhaps not,' I say doubtfully. 'It's my birthday and I'm having a party.'

'Oh. What a bloody fiftieth birthday present.'

'You mean it *is* ALS.'

'Yes, or a strange kind of Parkinson's.'

When we drive towards Stockholm, whirling snow is falling. Visibility is poor and the summer tyres only just keep the car on the road.

Home at last, I fall on to my bed and sleep heavily. Through my appointment at the hairdresser's.

Wake up two hours before the party.

Decision: don't say anything to anyone about today. Have fun and postpone the pain until tomorrow.

Scallops on skewers.

Terrine with salmon, spinach and sage.

Marinated fillet of lamb with plum chutney.

Potato frittata.

A little pannacotta with blueberries to follow.

Masses of wine, of course.

Mimmi and Lusse have organized everything.

And I enjoy the speeches. Which might have embarrassed me otherwise.

This evening I enjoy myself and laugh. Carry my secret and toss my head.

Glasses clink and my faithful friend Lars stands up. He expresses himself well, is amusing and serious: 'In hard times one makes friends for life. It's then that our mask falls and we get close to each other.'

We dance all night. And the music is loud.

It's my party.

A birthday party for everyone.

But for me, it is so much more.

At four o'clock my right leg can't cope any more.

A birthday girl can lie down on the sofa if she wants to.

'Olle, it's out of the question for me to be a vegetable, totally paralysed in bed. At that point I'll take sleeping pills,' I say, upset after the appointment with the neuro-physiologist in Uppsala. Although I see that that course of action would be impossible: paralysed, how would I swallow the pills? If anyone helped me, they'd be charged with murder.

'You can't do something like that to the children, especially the boys. You must give the medics a chance to help.'

He tells me that the neurologist has said that ALS patients are given morphine in the final phase. The thought gives me strength.

'Will you be ashamed of me when I'm sitting in a wheelchair with my tongue hanging out?'

The question is ridiculous, but necessary. He replies that he will never be ashamed and that he can wipe his Ussepusse's bottom.

It is Walpurgis Eve, the traditional spring festival.

'It may be the last time I experience the spring,' I say to my neighbour. I know he won't think I'm being silly. Because it may be true. But to see something for the last time can be as intense as seeing it for the first time. I enjoy the scillas, crocuses, and chaffinches, and I laugh at the wagtail's funny little nodding head.

But today I'm tired. We are due at Saltsjöbaden for a party. It's a burden, but I have to go.

Olle has to help me on with my T-shirt. I manage to do up my bra myself by lying on the bed and pushing the eye to the hook with my sick hand in its cradle.

We leave in the car, and after two blocks I want to go home, but change my mind. I have to be sociable for Olle's sake. Simultaneously he says that he can go on his own. That dismays me. Would it be a relief for him to be spared having me there? To be spared having to drag around the skinny woman with the dangling right arm and the right leg that wants to bend outwards?

We have to wait outside the Karolinska Hospital,

because Olle has to deal with some paperwork. I sit in the passenger seat and stick my tongue out at the lipstick mirror in the sunvisor.

At first it feels ordinary but then I see the twitches. Fasciculations in the tongue indicate damage to the central nervous system. How interesting, I think, and study the grey mottled piece of flesh more closely. I can't feel anything. No bubbles, fishtails or bees, as I do in the rest of my body. Odd.

With that, terror creeps over me. My throat and tongue are sick too. The bulbar symptoms are starting. Tears start to flow, there are twitches in my eyes; the corners of my mouth are drawn downwards in that new, peculiar way.

I manage to pull myself together.

'Mustn't make the children anxious, Ulla-Carin.'

When we arrive at last, I open the car door with my left foot and feel a new heaviness in my right leg as I stand up. I limp towards the front door. Olle has already rushed in. Gustaf holds open the door for me. When I reach the doorstep I whimper: 'Are there a lot of stairs?'

'Just these,' replies Olle, a little ahead.

I am no further than the third step when I fall. Bang my right knee, and my hand, of course. It hurts so much that my blood pressure falls and I feel sick.

'Hey, watch your step, Usse,' says Olle, when he runs back on agile feet to help me, in response to Gustaf and Pontus's yells.

Lucky I had on my little hand-corset. Otherwise things would have been a lot worse.

That night at home, Gustaf is worried and lies very, very close.

'Mummy, I want your hand to get well. What if the left one gets sick too?'

'Then you'll have to help me even more,' I say, which is hardly consoling.

When I have put out the light, silent tears fall. They wet the pillowcase and I hug the cuddly leopard that Mimmi, my best friend, gave me.

Dream. It's warm outside. I'm driving an open silver car. It's not a convertible, but it has no windscreen. I'm leaning back and driving fast, very fast. I notice that I haven't fastened my seat-belt, but it doesn't matter. The speed and the air resistance press me backwards. There is a thumping in my body, and heavy pressure downwards on to the muscles of my backside. There is a bend in the road. I drive well, but end up on the verge, then manoeuvre the car back on to the right carriageway!

This year the spring feels different from others. I drive my new car with the automatic gears to the church at Östra Ryd. Pontus was christened here in 1993. I wore a terrible blue dress that Olle had bought. My bra was white and it showed through the chiffon. Today I have on beige Ralph Lauren chinos, done up with the help of the buttoner. The birches are dressed in green bridal veils, the birds are singing and chirping exactly as they should, and I am sitting in the pew by the font, crying.

I want my funeral to take place here.

I hope it will be at this time of year. Or perhaps when the autumn leaves are reddish-gold. Not in winter or in the heat of summer.

I want my ashes spread over the sea.

Hope that Olle will have the boat in the water by then.

Have read on some web-page that most die suffocated by their own mucus. Before I receive the final diagnosis from my neurologist I have read almost everything about amyotrophic lateral sclerosis, ALS.

Have found a way of washing my armpit, the left one: I pour liquid soap on to my left knee, position my armpit over it and rub it back and forth.

Today, 14 May 2003, is Doomsday. At three o'clock I'm sitting in Anne Zachau's office at the Karolinska Hospital in Solna.

'You look unhappy,' she says.

I answer something about my feeling serious.

She rambles on and on about the investigation having taken a long time, but it has been difficult. I consider interrupting but realize she is building up to something significant.

'As you have already realized, you have ALS,' she says.

And this is true. I knew I was right. Nonetheless, I ask her to continue, and she talks about difficulties in diagnosing, prescribing medicines, reacting, informing . . . I ruffle my feathers. There is a creeping sensation beneath my skin. What else does she know about me and my future? They look so impassive, she and Olle. He is leaning back a little in the visitor's chair, his left leg crossed over the right, and he nods politely.

How will he and my small boys manage? I'm hurting him, I think. Panic urgently insists that I get out of the room. I fetch a mug of lukewarm hospital water. Composed again.

'If you were me, what would you do now?'

'I'd travel to Hawaii,' she says. 'But, of course, you have a family and I haven't. Your family is your Hawaii.'

'Although it's terribly sad to be terminally ill and have children, I also feel so rich,' I say. I am fulfilled through my daughters and my sons.

'Have you a friend for me?' I wonder. 'Someone like me who is in the same situation?'

'Ulla-Carin,' she replies, 'not just at the moment. I haven't any other patient as bright and gifted as you.'

Vanity allows me to feel flattered. She explains that it is often high-achievers who become ill. She tells me, too, how the respiratory muscles become affected and, in the end, paralysed.

'How long will I live?'

'I don't know. It depends on when your respiratory system stops working.'

'"When?" You say "when" and not "if"?'

'Yes. You ask straight questions, so you get straight answers.'

Perhaps I'm unfeeling. It is as if I haven't the strength to cry. The corner of my mouth quivers when she looks at Olle and says how difficult it can be for the family.

It makes me sad to cause him pain.

I have to show her my tongue. 'It's so ugly,' I whisper stupidly. She does not see any special fasciculations, nerve twitches. I have to hop on my left leg. That's all right. Then on the right. I can't.

She does not contradict me when I say that the illness seems to progress fairly rapidly.

Ring my elder daughter.

'Ulrica, it's the worst possible news. I've got ALS. The doctor told me.'

'Mummy, I'd already worked that out.'

Yes, most of the people around me have, and it is three months since the Swiss doctor didn't protest when I suggested that it was ALS. It has taken such a long time to confirm the diagnosis.

'When did you know?'

'I was sitting in a park, studying with some friends. It was the first day of spring. The sunshine was strong and my eyes weren't used to it. Out of the blue, one of my friends, a medical student, said: "Look, Ulle, here's a disease similar to your mother's." I read the text she gave me. Medical English. What are "motor-neurones"? Oh yes . . . "Often starts with one of the hands. Spreads. All patients dead within ten years. Most common among men and in Asian countries. Paralysis, but the perception of touch is unaffected. The intellect remains intact." I got an icy feeling inside. It's this. I know it.

'Back home I searched on the net. A doctor in Umeå: "The worst diagnosis one can give a patient. Fifty per cent die within eighteen months of diagnosis."

'Mummy, I know everything, and nothing is ever going to be the same again.'

I put down the receiver and ring Carin. Engaged. I try again and when she replies she's in a terrible state. Ulrica got in first.

My mother, aged eighty-one, says I'm so young that the scientists will come up with some effective medication.

She probably knows it's already too late. But I agree, to comfort her.

You won't help me by crying. I can't comfort you. Perhaps the time for crying will come for me too. But at present I'm too tired.

When I get home from work, he is sitting there, he who used to be my comforter, in my chair under my birch tree in my garden. The birch is shimmeringly green now, in May. It is still chilly, but sunny too. At night the water is alight with the full moon. It is a slow spring and for me that feels good.

He comes towards me and his face is wet with tears. He comes like a dog with its tail between its legs, and whimpers. Does he want me to scratch him, to stroke him? I drag myself out of the car and say, without meeting the look on that wet face, that this isn't the time for tears.

'How will I cope if you start crying over me now? Perhaps you'll be disappointed if I live for years.'

'Somebody has to die in order that the rest of us should value life more,' says Virginia Woolf, as played by Nicole Kidman in *The Hours*. The film deals a lot with the right to choose. Richie, sick with Aids, keeps himself alive only so that he does not disappoint Clarissa. He feels there is no dignity in his life.

It's a new way of being. At this moment I have a sense of the present. I feel I've won greater understanding. Participation, but also outsidership. A feeling of being chosen. Strange and a little crazy?

I am the one who will go first.

Nurse Margaretha has been the head of the Karolinska ALS team since the mid-sixties. She meets me without fear. She wants me to ask things. I feel an impulse to tease her, so I ask her to tell me stuff instead. She says that the ALS team consists of a counsellor, a physiotherapist, a dietician, a nurse and a doctor. In that order. I have to ask about the illness. She is clearly afraid of saying too much. I hear her say that I have classic ALS: it begins on one side, then spreads, progressing with its destruction at an even rate. I suggest that surely it is possible to work out mathematically when I'm going to die.

'But your having ALS doesn't necessarily mean you'll die of it. Something else might happen to you,' she says.

Funnily enough, this disappoints me. If I have a terminal illness I may as well die of it.

She states that I already have some difficulty in breathing because my stomach muscles are deteriorating. I just have time to think that my stomach is still flat and hard – vanity is a weighty part of my almost fifty-five kilos worth of body – before I am blowing into an apparatus that measures the capacity of the lungs. 'We have to have a measurement to start from.'

Eighty per cent. An excellent result. Later on, she says, I'll need a ventilator, a mask to breathe into every day. I'll have to use it before I make any effort and before I go to bed. 'It can be tough at night otherwise. One breathes differently at night.'

I don't want to understand what the woman is talking about.

It's 6 June, Sweden's National Day, and the boys and I are having breakfast on the balcony. It seems that it's going to be a fantastic Whitsun holiday. I'm going to tell them the difficult news now.

'My doctor says that my hand will never be all right.'

'But the doctor said it was because you fell off the horse,' says Pontus. 'That it might be all right.'

'It isn't going to get better. It's going to get worse. It's already started in my right leg. Have you noticed?'

One of them has.

'Won't you be able to walk in the future?'

'No, I'm going to sit in a wheelchair. Will you run races with me in it?' I wonder, laughing.

Gustaf is perplexed. He looks at me angrily and accusingly: 'D'you think this is funny, or what?'

'No, it's sad and tiresome to have a serious illness.'

'Mummy, I don't want you to die before me,' Pontus bursts out.

'Oh, yes, my boy, I'm going to. That's God's plan, and

that's the way it has to be. You're going to grow up and have children.'

I get out the cuddly toys, who have also been listening, and ask if they've understood this matter of Mummy's illness. It seems so, because they say nothing. I tell them and the boys to ask questions, if they wonder about anything.

Breakfast is over.

I dream weird things.

The letters on my script run when the studio light is switched on.

I give the usual greeting 'Good evening,' and discover that the script is made of pistachio-green marzipan.

It sticks to my fingers in the heat.

The letters are written in pink icing and everything is melting as though it were a painting by Salvador Dalí.

How can I be dreaming this – again – three years after my last news show?

I rush down a spiral staircase and hear editor Ingemar Odlander's stern voice. 'Where the hell is Ulla-Carin?'

The makeup girl is at the ready with the powder compact and I know I haven't got a chance.

Will never make it.

Odlander's voice is distant.

Can't find my way.

Lost.

Creep through different rooms.

See faces I recognize.

No one sees me.

'Where is the presenter?'

Always in a hurry and always have been.

A roe deer seeks shelter in the beech woods. Hides.

Flees at the slightest suspicion of danger.

That's me.

(Under pressure.)

My daughters.

(Perpetual guilt.)

My sons.

My husband.

(Always preoccupied.)

The studio.

Controlled.

Collected.

I have been driven by adrenaline. I have sought chaos.

Hunger has been my fuel.

Flight my companion.

In the pursuit of being good enough. Of being acknowledged.

How was it possible?

'It'll be better tomorrow.'

'I'll do it later.'

'It'll sort itself out later.'

'First I'm just going to . . .'

It was not possible.

I believe that stress and strain have made me vulnerable to the illness.

An ALS-patient has to economize with her resources: they aren't renewed. After one day of effort you need, perhaps, two days of rest. It's a question of finding a balance. Rest and activity have to balance each other on the scales. Strong feelings are a strain and make the patient worse. Better to live calmly.

'Who is your typical patient?' I ask Nurse Margaretha.

Her reply comes straightaway: 'Well-educated, highly intelligent, with great integrity. Seldom overweight or careless with themselves. Often sporty. Eighty per cent of my patients are what one usually calls type-A individuals. They are high achievers with integrity who make huge demands on themselves.'

As she tells me this I, who am terminally ill, am vain enough to feel proud.

To think I belong to this group!

She tells me about a father of two children. He was my age and had children like my boys.

He brought them with him to the surgery so that they could follow his decline, his journey towards the end.

I think it *is* rather like a journey. I can choose which compartment to sit in, which people to meet. It sounds almost pleasant.

I wrote this on Crete, just south of Heraklion. It was June 2003. When I wanted to lever myself out of the hotel bathtub, I couldn't. Olle was out, and I could cry for as long as I liked. It was the first time I checked the muscles of my right leg. They were thinner than those of the left. I'm not going to compare them any more.

Pontus, my elder son, is ten years and nine months old. These are his thoughts on 16 July 2003. He's agreed that you and I can read what he's written in his diary:

Mummy has an illness which causes the nerves to make her muscles weaker. She has got it in her right arm, leg and left arm. I feel sorry for her. Mummy can't walk up stairs, carry, run, jump, swim, wash her hair, etc. She doesn't work as much. Mummy can't get out of bed as fast. She feels sorry for me. I just think it's fun to help her. I want her to write a diary because then I can read it when she's dead. It's lucky that Mimmi is here, she helps Mummy a lot. I have dreamt that I was a doctor and that there was a way you could remove this illness by operation. Then I would do that on her. I want to know more about Mummy's illness. Why not get hold of a robot arm. I've seen it on TV. They're steered by the muscles in the shoulder. I think that this is a good idea. Mummy can't walk long distances. Mummy is clever at writing with her left hand. I love my Mummy anyway.

I have to take each day as it comes, they say.

I wake up beside the father of my sons and sniff his smell a little. But always with that stab of inadequacy. My inadequacy. Although I am, of course, to take the day as it comes. I am happy that I succeed in levering myself up in bed, shuffling to the loo and pulling down my pyjama trousers. I can still wipe myself. It is still only the twisting movement and the tweezer grip that my left hand has difficulty with.

I prepare two ham sandwiches and a cup of coffee. It goes down the wrong way twice. It's embarrassing in front of Olle, and my inadequacy gnaws at me again. Coffee dribbles out of the corners of my mouth.

The geese are flocking. It is 23 July. The young birds are preparing to fly south. It is calm and the sun is hanging heavy over the grove, which is starting to grow too tall. But at the same time it affords protection against the west-north-westerly, which sometimes shrieks over the fields and meadows.

The dogdays have arrived and almost a year has passed since I discovered the hollow between my index finger and thumb.

Every year I feel a little sad when the geese gather. It's the same this time. But more so now.

A diver bird calls, desolate but majestic, over the slow swell of dusk. In July the sun has reached the islet's southern headland. In August there is space for it in the gap between the tops of the pines on the other side. The gulls settle and are only tempted by Östen Bolin's rowing-boat, which is ploughing through the water. Now he throws away the small fry, and the peace is shattered by a cacophony of screeches. His wife Elsa-Lena is waiting with the glowing hot sauna. Their daughters crowd round the zinc tub, which will soon be filled with perch, pike, turbot and perhaps even a pike-perch.

It is at our neighbours', the Bolins', that my brother and I, as children, seek our refuge for warmth and simple caring. Not much is lovelier than Elsa-Lena's rhubarb cordial seen against the light, just brought up from the earth cellar. We find the cardamom rusks in a biscuit tin wedged on to the top shelf. At the Bolins', life is wrapped up and protected against the hard south-westerly. While the dogs' ears are pressed against their skulls as they sniff into the headwind at our home, Anita stands and rinses lustre cream shampoo out of Brita's hair, sheltered from the wind behind their cottage. There's a tingly feeling in the pit of my stomach as I see her take a dollop of the creamy shampoo and slowly massage it into her little sister's hair. Now she is pumping water into the yellow enamel jug and mixing it to the right temperature for rinsing. There is a calm and tenderness about her that I have only seen when Daddy, under the influence of his evening drink, caresses his pointer.

At five in the afternoon we hear the horn of the Volvo and we stand to attention and wait. From the boot we lift wooden crates with soft drinks, soda water, tonic and class IIA beer. I, the smallest, hurry to sort them into rows in the nooks beneath the jetty where we do the washing-up. We have already laid the table and scraped the new potatoes, and now Daddy mixes the drinks and Mummy pours dry-roasted peanuts into a bowl, whose pattern is said to be made from grains of rice.

The schnapps is ice-chilled as usual, on this Thursday evening, and all four of us sing that we'll take a sip to wet our lip. As usual, I am embarrassed by it and Mummy's way of getting us into the mood, but the orangeade is good. Yes, Mummy, of course, and yes, please, to more of that oily herring from Strååth's fish shop by the river in Kristinehamn. But best of all are the prawns crammed with roe, and when Mummy sings about Mr Boll the frog and Kalle Stropp to the music of the accordion. Daddy is stroking his dog Raff, and we have our pyjamas on. I am carried away by the song, which takes me to India on a seagull's back. Mummy has made up her own version of it. Her dark alto doesn't reach to the top of the Himalayas, but I'm put to bed in contentment under the red silk coverlet, and the hot grey stones at the foot of the bed weigh me to sleep without any amen.

Today I read what I had written to Carin. I began to cry when I reached 'amen'.

What have I done wrong, to be struck down by a terminal illness?

Why am I being punished?

After the diagnosis, shame strikes me.

I have been too lucky. And not thankful enough for it.

A connection still exists between illness and punishment for sin: the English word 'pain' comes from the Greek '*poine*', which means punishment.

Deep inside me is the idea that one can be punished with illness.

And that everything will be all right if only one is kind, rosy-cheeked and doesn't put one's foot in it.

'Glad and good shall a person be whilst awaiting death.' This maxim was embroidered on a wall-hanging in Greatgrandmother's kitchen.

To whom have I not been grateful enough?

At our old nursery school, there was a boy who used to build churches with the wooden bricks. His mother is a vicar and I reach her on her mobile.

We send text messages during the summer.

'We pray for you every day in our prayer group.'

Strangely, it embarrasses me that she prays for me.

And a whole group too.

What on earth do they say?

Ought *I* to pray?

I sit in the deck-chair and gaze at the power in the sea.

It gives me strength.

Is sitting and watching the waves the same as praying for strength?

Is it good enough?

When we leave the beach in Ystad I see how three wind-power stations coalesce into one for the blink of an eye.

The wind-power stations act as a navigation beacon and I make my way towards the one that is furthest away.

I wade through poppies, with their skirts of crumpled silk, and flick at dandelion clocks. Beyond roars the sea.

Here is my road now.
My navigation beacon, which I must follow.
And the sea can be my altar.

Between our ears there is a grey lump that weighs about a kilo: the brain. It is our last unexplored continent. We still do not know much about how it works. But we know when it doesn't work. According to the Brain Fund, a million Swedes are suffering from some form of disease or disturbance of the brain's function. Six hundred have ALS. Compare that figure with the one hundred thousand stroke patients.

ALS stands for amyotrophic lateral sclerosis. The motor nerve cells – meaning those that supply the muscles – die in the brain, in the brainstem and in the outer part of the spinal cord. Lateral means 'at the side of'. The nerve cells are replaced with connective tissue, sclerosis. The muscles, '*myosis*' in Greek, do not receive impulses from the nerves, become weak and atrophy. '*Trophi*' is the Greek word for 'nourishment'. In this case the nourishment in question is nerve signals. 'Atrophy' is the opposite: it means something is missing.

The lack of nerve impulses leads to the wasting of the muscles which are controlled by will.

We cannot control the heart, but we can hold our breath. So the lungs are controlled by the nerves that are knocked out by ALS.

ALS patients die when their breathing is put out of action.

The summer of 2003 will perhaps be my last. In any case it will be the last when I'm standing on my own two legs. We buy a beach chair and I have to be lifted out of it. One evening my sons, daughters, a boyfriend and I play Kubb, a game from Gotland, in the yard. I sway and strut about like a drunk but succeed in casting two bullseyes with my left hand, which is weak too now.

Olle gives me a sunset as a present on my saint's day. He chops a gap in the bushes where the sun goes down over the beech woods, and the shadows get longer.

My strength is ebbing away and a summer cold gives the illness a push forward.

I feel great sadness and cry buckets.

Friends comfort me and say they are sure they have heard of people who have had ALS for ten years. But how can I cope with feeling like this for ten more years? I know that my time will not be that long.

In August I visit my neurologist Anne Zachau again. Mimmi is with me. I tape the entire conversation.

Death is so important that one has the right to be told things straight.

'I'm a journalist. I'm used to working to a deadline. What have I got to work to now?'

'You want to know when you're going to die?'

'Hmm.'

'Do you think I can tell?'

'Yes. You must know whether it will be five years, three or less?'

'Well, I don't think it'll be as much as five years, or even three. Rather, one or two. But it's a question nobody wants to answer. When you ask a straight question you put me in a difficult position. But you have the right to know.

'It depends on respiratory function. If you're going to die of ALS and not of anything else beforehand, it will be because respiration fails. This is irrespective of whether or not you can move your legs or swallow.

'You may have had this for three years. When you first notice a weakening, you have already lost eighty per cent of the nerve fibres in that muscle.

'The cause is unknown. It might be that a virus has lain dormant in the body. It is often a common virus. Free radicals have also been mentioned.

'The patients I meet have often been healthy, remarkably healthy, and very active. Many sportsmen have been struck down by ALS. That doesn't mean that you'll get it *because* you play baseball in the USA or ice hockey in Sweden or paddle a canoe.

'It isn't fair that you can become ill when you have lived a healthy life. It probably depends on your body and your genes. How vulnerable they are.'

This is according to Snow White, Anne Zachau, my neurologist.

The same day, Nurse Margaretha gives me a breathing test. In June my lung capacity was eighty per cent, which she told me was good. Today I only achieve sixty-three per cent.

'We'll see that you get a ventilator,' says Nurse Margaretha, and dries my tears.

The next day I don't get out of my pyjamas until just before the boys arrive home from school.

I have now become a case for the municipal bureaucracy.

One in a stack of files in a civil servant's office.

'It's not possible to get help just like that. That wouldn't look good, would it?'

'But she has to have help now!' says Mimmi, on the telephone.

'It just so happens that it's still the holidays.'

'She has two small boys at home and she's begun to fall over.'

The next day I am given emergency home care while I wait for the decision about a personal home carer.

The bristles scratch my childish skin, turning it pink. Granny, in silk blouse, grey skirt and pearls, bends down and brushes me. She pats me here and there with the brush.

'My little pet has clothes with spots on.'

She brushes back and forth.

'And now she's got clothes with stripes.'

I laugh until I choke when she rinses soapy clothes off me. Huge drops fall from the shower, heavy and slow.

This was long before she faded away in the geriatric ward in Kristinehamn.

'Call me when you need me,' says Lisa now, and I balance carefully on the edge of the bath. Get hold of the shower's wall-fitting and lift my right leg with its lead fetter. It gives way and I fall into the rosemary-scented bubbles with a bump, hurting my coccyx. But the warmth is immediate and comforting and I lower my head under the water.

Lisa rubs my back with the special flannel from the chemist's, and I try to lift my paralysed right arm so that she can reach my armpit. She is forty-six and likes caring for the aged and infirm.

The day after, Aden from Somalia turns up. He is black and wears a cap. I stammer something about planning to take a shower and am told that he has already showered two women today and is good at blow-drying hair. I realize that I will have to get used to it and start to enjoy the thought of testing myself.

It's perfectly OK.

The decision about personal home care still hasn't come through. The illness takes over more and more and now I hardly dare go up or down the stairs alone. I have to think 'backwards' so that I don't fall headlong when the jangling in my nerves upsets my balance.

The Karolinska Hospital exerts pressure, but it doesn't help. I'm stuck in the queue and everyone works as fast as they can.

The council has to decide and after that the social-security office.

Forms are filled in at terrific speed. And I write a covering letter:

REASONS FOR NEEDING A CARER

I am suffering from classic ALS. It is fast and aggressive. A year ago I was working full-time as a TV journalist. Today I am not only incapable of taking care of the simplest household chores but am also incapable of taking care of my personal hygiene in a satisfactory way.

I have two children at home, aged eight and ten, and a husband who works full-time.

Up to now, the illness has led to total paralysis of my right arm, acute reduction in and weakening of the left hand, drop-foot and stiffness in my right leg, and the beginning of the same in the left. I can, with great difficulty, walk five metres. My breathing capacity is decreasing, according to the same linear principle, and I am shortly to be tested for a ventilator. Since the ALS has also attacked my tongue, I have difficulty in talking and swallowing.

The illness gives rise to spastic spasms and nervous twitches throughout my body.

WHAT I NEED HELP WITH
I need help to live what is left of my life in a tolerable way.

This means, among other things, help with breakfast, personal hygiene, dressing, making the bed, getting around, cooking and laundry. In addition I would like the carers to help me at the computer and in other intellectual work, which remains my main interest.

The above takes place from early in the morning until late afternoon.

After that, I need help with preparing another meal, various household tasks, intellectual work, personal hygiene and undressing until my husband arrives home in the evening. I should stress that my problems get worse during the course of the day.

Furthermore, I need support and help in contacting all the medical professionals connected to my case.

This means that I need help twelve hours a day during weekdays, or one full-time and one part-time home carer. During weekends my need is less when my husband is not on call. At the moment I estimate that I need help for about six hours a day at weekends, when he is at home.

I want to give the strength that I have left to my four children, of whom two are young.

Täby, 26 August 2003
Ulla-Carin Lindquist

A couple of weeks later a team of people who will decide my case arrive at my home to discuss *in situ* the help I need.

They sit in the living-room: an assessor from the social-security office and one from the council, the counsellor from the hospital and Mimmi.

'We have to know exactly how long it takes you to carry out different activities.'

'How do you mean?'

'How long does it take you to get dressed?'

'But I'm unable to get dressed.'

'About how long?'

'I really can't do it. Didn't you read the letter I wrote?'

The woman from the council has not seen it. The one from the social-security office has a spare copy with her.

'That's not enough. We have to have a time.'

'You're joking.'

'No.'

'But I can't. The home carer dresses me. I can't put on a pair of trousers without falling over.'

It goes on like that for a while. I am classified, weighed, evaluated.

Neither the council nor the social-security office has realized what they are up against in Mimmi. She gets angry: 'Do you want to know how long it takes for her to change a tampon?'

Embarrassment.

It becomes clear that they want to make a show of their power. 'There are regulations.'

'What are you waiting for? Here's a doctor's certificate that explains everything. The occupational-therapist's analysis. Don't you see? She can't even pick her nose!'

'Who makes the decisions for the council?' I ask.

'I do.'

'Just you?'

'Yes.'

'So, decide now!'

'That's not the way things work.'

'Then decide tomorrow.'

'That's not the way things work either. I can't make a decision until next week.'

Then the lady from the social-security office, who is more experienced, changes sides: 'I shall recommend that Ulla-Carin gets the help she's applying for.'

Early the next morning, when I am lying in bed, waiting for the home carer, the telephone rings.

'Hallo, I'm calling from the council. You've been granted the carer you applied for.'

Yet again I receive confirmation that one needs the gift of the gab, to have a tongue in one's head and to be thick-skinned to penetrate officialdom.

How would Aden from Somalia cope if he was in my position?

The laughter just bubbles out. I try to stop it, press my hand to my lips but a cascade of *café au lait* sprays over the table.

'I-I-I said paren'-teasher meeting . . . paren'- pa'en-'easher mee'ing . . . is what I said,' I stammer. In the end 'parent-teacher meeting' comes out with an American drawl and I succeed in telling him that Class 4A has a meeting on Tuesday.

'What Nurse Margaretha in the ALS team says is probably right, that you may laugh for no apparent reason. But that can be amusing,' says Olle, and looks as though he thinks quite the opposite.

'Slapstick, I vashue slapstick mush more nowawaysh,' I laugh until I choke and start to cough. The absurd can often be comical.

'Olle, give me two minutes,' I beg, and explain slowly, drawling, but articulating as well as I can, 'OK, I have an illness that embodies aspects similar to incurable cancer.'

Here I guffaw again.

'"Embodies"! Maybe I should try "has similarities to"

instead,' I say when the attack of laughter has died down.

I am going to die of ALS, if nothing unpredictable happens. There are two roads I can take. One is to lie down, be bitter and wait. The other is to make something worthwhile of the misfortune. See it in a positive light, however banal that sounds. My road is the second. I have to live in the immediate present. There is no bright future for me. But there is a bright present. Children live like this. Only for the present. Nothing coming afterwards. Therefore I laugh like a child. Uncontrollably.

The whole of my adult life I have thought, it will be all right in the end. I have to do this first, then it will be all right.

But this way of thinking is no longer possible. The strange thing is that nowadays, when I am terminally ill, I feel moments of great joy, such as I have hardly ever felt before. Happiness has never been a constant for me, but now it is becoming one.

That's why I laugh.

And if it has anything to do with bulbar paralysis, then it is a blessing that comes with ALS.

My words get stuck in my nose. It feels as though my palate has been cleft. As though the soft palate is slackening. My tongue looks a little furry and I can no longer put out the tip like a snake. Instead, there is a snakepit in it. Nerve twitchings in my tongue. And my mouth snuffles forth unintelligible sounds. It is as though a gramophone record is being played at the wrong speed.

ALS has deprived me of the spoken word. My speech. The tool of my trade. Today nobody has understood what I said. Fury.

In my head my thoughts are clearer than ever before. I hear my voice inside me. A melody and an intonation that were an important part of my job. But now my voice passes the larynx, the ALS filter, and only an inarticulate sound comes out. Like a braying donkey.

ALS has already deprived me of my right hand. It lies at eternal rest. Bluish like a well-hung fillet of beef. The left has three fingers with the strength to write on the computer. But they are stiff and get cramp.

'Why couldn't you have given me two lame legs

instead? Dear God, be kind to my three fingers and my tongue.'

ALS is a spiteful, mocking laugh.

There is no cure for ALS but there is a drug that – at best – may help the patient live a little longer. It is called Rilutek, and the active ingredient is riluzole.

In an experiment a group of patients were given Rilutek and compared with a control group who received a placebo. The patients were monitored for between twelve and twenty-one months. The Rilutek group lived on average three months longer.

In the official Swedish medicine manual it says: 'There is no evidence that riluzole has any therapeutic effect on motor functions, lung function, fasciculations, muscle power and motor symptoms. Riluzole has not been shown to be effective in the later stages of ALS.'

What does that mean?

No more than that a patient may survive an extra three months if she starts early with the medicine and carries on for a long time, at least a year. It says nothing about the quality of the possible period of life-extension.

It seems pointless.

Three months: that's nothing, I think, when the tablets make me tired in the beginning.

So I stop.

For three days.

Then I dare not continue without them.

'Studies do not explain how the drug works for the individual patient,' says the neurologist.

She tells me that Rilutek may protect the brain from attacks by glutamate, a transmitter substance in the brain. Too much damages the nerve cells, and they believe that patients with ALS have too much.

I read about the short lifespan of those who have my type of ALS.

And time takes on another perspective. Another significance.

Three more months with the children!

If only, if only.

To believe in medicine would be the height of folly, if it were not an even greater folly not to believe in it.

Marcel Proust

I am not my body.

I am in it.

It is sick, but my spirit is healthy.

My self is my soul and it is strong.

This suffering can be my strength.

Primordial strength. As when a child's head rotates out of the uterus.

I know that it will end. Make myself strong. Calm.

Life is full of new beginnings.

Laughter is a deliverance. Disarming. It keeps danger at bay. Both aspects of a theatre mask: one happy, one sad. A fragile thread between tragedy and comedy.

Never before has such a lovely woman crossed my threshold, and she is carrying ten roses, the colour of apricots and the size of a fist.

The atmosphere is charged. This woman has been recently widowed. She has four children. The eldest is eleven. Her husband died of ALS. He did not even reach the age of fifty.

I contacted her to learn how she and her husband prepared the children, but first I want to know about the course of the illness. I get to know, in detail, and I regret it.

First he noticed weakness creeping up on him and one day he was unable to lift weights. My clothes-peg was the equivalent. After the diagnosis he went for alternative medical care abroad and came home with boxes of dried lizards and snakes' eyes. His wife made a concoction of them, which filled the whole house with a new smell. She gave him some to drink, and masses of vitamins, antioxidants and creatine, which is good for the muscles.

The doctor gave him a year. He lived twice as long.

When he had his first bout of pneumonia, the doctors asked her, 'Do you want us to give your husband antibiotics or do you want him to be allowed to pass away?'

She was angry so the doctors treated him. After that he survived five more bouts of pneumonia. He died of the after-effects of the seventh.

The children who asked most questions and helped her most have so far coped best. The children who avoided everything are anxious and insecure.

'Answer all questions and let the children be part of it,' is her simple advice.

The woman with the roses sat on my sofa for three hours.

She said that the children cannot remember a healthy daddy, only a sick one.

None of them can imagine that the suntanned man on the ski slope in the photograph in the hall is the same daddy as the one they remember.

At Vrinnevi Hospital in Norrköping there is a special children's trauma team. Therapists explain to me how they believe one should deal with children when a parent has a terminal illness.

'The children must be allowed to know. It can be one or both parents who do the explaining. Sometimes it is good to let a doctor give the information and let the children have a chance to ask questions. They often do so directly. Some children may be in denial and not want to hear. Then you must back off and try again. Say, for example, "We must talk about this. It will only take five minutes," then start to explain again.

'The situation you parents are facing causes stress for you all. What you have to tell them is the worst thing a parent can say to their child. But the child must have a chance to begin to process what is happening.

'Since your speech is already so poor it is important that you do this as soon as possible. Show the children that you are sad so that you allow them the chance to be sad. Explain why you are sad too.

'Explaining prepares the children and arms them for what is to come,' say Ken Chesterton and Lars Widén, psychotherapists in the children's trauma team. 'But both parents must agree on how they are going to go about it.'

'Mummy, are you going to talk about that illness again now? You know already that you're just getting badder, so why are you sad?' says Gustaf, who will soon be nine.

And the day after, when he can't grasp what I say, 'You could at least *try* to speak so that we understand.'

I laugh and promise I will.

When the children have left for school I dial the number of our country cottage. I want to hear myself on the answering-machine. As I sounded when I was healthy. I ring four times.

Pontus wants us to create a blink language.

'Three blinks are "I love you."'

He blinks three times. I blink three times at him and have difficulty in holding back my tears.

'Mummy, two blinks mean "yes" and one long one "no".'

He says we're going to practise a lot, and I blink twice.

Sweden's minister of foreign affairs, Anna Lindh, is dead, stabbed in a department store. The planet Mars stares at me with its single eye in the clear September night. The prime minister Göran Persson reads a poem by Tomas Tranströmer: 'Inside you, vault beyond vault opens out towards infinity.'

The EU commissioner Margot Wallström speaks about the grief that wells up as water does when thin ice cracks. Pontus's eyes are like the first ice of winter, thin and transparent, cracked by the weight of the realization that I'm going to die.

All these sunny days that should make it easier to deliver sad tidings.

'Today is a good day to tell them. We're both here and it's lovely weather.'

Yes, it's undeniably easier like this.

'What you have to tell them now is the worst thing a parent can say to their child. But the child must have a chance to begin to process this,' said the psychotherapists in Norrköping.

We sit on the double bed and I tell them I'm glad that Mimmi and Ingrid are my carers and that they help me.

'Soon I'll need even more help, because I'm just getting sicker.'

(Beloved Gustaf, you frown with irritation and say, 'Are you going to talk about that illness again?')

We tell them that the hospital has measured my breathing, that it is only fifty-four per cent now, that it will become even worse and that it is hard to live with only a little air. Pontus says, 'You know you're going to get a machine to breathe into,' and I tell them that that will only help a little and that, anyway, the breathing muscles are breaking down.

'You said your lungs wouldn't get sick,' remembers Gustaf.

'No, she said her heart,' Pontus corrects him.

I tell them that ALS is among the worst illnesses that a person can get. Olle says that it isn't infectious and can't be inherited. I say I have the best doctor in Sweden and the most wonderful family in the world. Olle and I start to cry and –

'What's it going to be like in a year?'

Emptiness. Time stops. My throat tightens. Gustaf's eyes are like ponds and he is waiting.

'I'll probably be dead.'

Pontus bursts into tears and dives down beside me in bed while Gustaf remains in the chair by the window.

Behind him a westerly wind is blowing. The sailing-boats are travelling north with the wind side-on towards the harbour in Viggbyholm. The rosehips glow scarlet.

'Now I want to tell you about the stone age!' Gustaf says.

He explains in detail about food hollows and flints.

Pontus continues to lie with me, gazing into my eyes, close. When we have learnt how people lived six thousand years ago, Pontus cycles to his friend Marcus, and a little later he is sitting on the hilltop looking out to sea with a bag of cheese-and-onion crisps.

My carer Ingrid has just helped me out of bed, fed me, showered me and massaged anti-ageing cream with St John's wort into my face.

I received a delivery of new anti-wrinkle creams last week at the same time as Mimmi bought me a new blue-grey designer T-shirt.

Before, when I was healthy, I would have thought it was verging on indecency for a terminally ill person to spend money on frivolity and finery.

Now it feels more important than ever to look fresh. Every morning I want to have Bulgari Eau Fraîche in the hollow of my throat, my eyebrows plucked, my legs shaved and my toenails varnished.

'It doesn't matter what you look like, as long as you're good!'

My grandma Sigrid, who sprang from a family of churchmen in Värmland, looks at me sternly. I am standing in her room and gazing at my reflection in the mirror. The sun is shining into the room, which faces the garden with Gravensteiner and Astrakan apple trees.

Grandma always wears a checked pinafore and her front teeth stick out, being aired.

'If the cock crows and the wind changes, you will stay like that,' she says, when I squint, and I believe her.

The royal family hang on the wall in her bedroom. When Anders Franzén salvages the man-o'-war, the *Vasa*, I am given a souvenir coin made of rolled gold. My grandma shows me that when one reverses the year 1961 it becomes the same number, and we sit at her sewing-table turning the coin over and over. I am allowed to choose whether the doll's dress is to be pink or light blue. She makes it with puff sleeves, smocking and feather-stitch embroidery. The mother-of-pearl buttons have four holes, and as a bonus the doll without a name is given a lace petticoat.

Whenever we go to buy plain buns we walk east along Södra Staketgatan. There, the houses are timbered, with loft passageways, and I do not know anybody. We turn off towards Österlånggatan where there is a stench of coal and rancid margarine. As we approach Knutsson's bakery, the air is redolent with smells, and the sound of the doorbell makes my mouth water so much that I almost dribble. On the way home, we go to the dairy on the corner. Today there is a party and there is a clatter on the marble counter as the assistant pours three measures of cream. Back in Grandma's kitchen, I perch at the kitchen table and eat a bun with goat's milk butter and drink raspberry cordial without slurping.

Gustaf comes and stands beside my desk.

'Do you write all the time, Mummy?'

'It takes such a long time,' I reply. 'I only write with two fingers now.'

'Mummy, I'm a miniature human being.'

'What?'

'You're big and I'm little.'

'No, Gustaf. You're big. You have your whole life in front of you. The future. Now it's me who's getting smaller.'

'Mummy, every second is a life,' he says gently.

'What did you say?'

'Every second is a life.'

'Where have you heard that?'

'Nowhere. I just made it up.'

And he carries on: 'You have hundreds of thousands of lives left, Mummy.'

'Every second is a life,' I echo.

Pontus ponders how he can develop our blink language.

Up to now we have signals for 'yes', 'no', and 'I love you' which can go a long way, if the questions are straight and come one at a time. The last signal, three blinks, needs no question.

'Mummy,' he says, and rolls his eyes. 'This means "pocket money".'

He rolls his eyes again.

'Pocket money!'

'Yes, but it's me who won't be able to talk later on,' I protest.

'But it's fun,' he replies, and rolls his eyes.

I blink twice in reply and Pontus fetches my purse.

There is a lot that's new for all four children.

Ulrica, who is twenty-three and has just passed her first-year exam in tax law, brushes mascara delicately on to my eyelashes.

She puts blusher on my cheeks and dabs cream on my spots.

Ties my hair up in a ponytail.

Smears cream on my hands.

Cleans my teeth carefully.

'You'll never smell bad, Mummy. I promise.'

She flosses my teeth.

'From now on I'm going to do for you what you did so many times for me.'

And then my despair wells up.

The dam bursts.

I cry into my elder daughter's stomach.

Later:

'I want you to tell me a place where I can meet you when you're dead, Mummy. Where you will be when I need you.'

I give her one.

'I know that you will always live in me. When I have problems or feel anxious, you will always be there to advise me, I know that,' says Ulrica, who was born between snowdrop and crocus.

I am now in the process of being adapted for disability. It is not only a matter of my own mental training but about steps that must be removed and the ones outside that must have a wheelchair ramp.

'We'll build the ramp straight out so the taxi service for the disabled can easily back in,' says the builder.

'Hell, no. Build it to the left so that Olle can still park in front,' I bleat. Then it won't be visible from the road, I think.

What a coward I am!

Do I despise the disabled? Am I ashamed? Do I despise weakness?

When Pontus arrives home with a new friend I ask if I can come in and say hallo.

'Of course, Mummy. Why are you asking?'

I'm asking because I want to protect him from being ashamed. But he is not ashamed. That idea does not exist in his world.

Sadly, I cannot deny the possibility that I would have been ashamed in his position.

While I devote myself to mental matters, the Täby council renovates the bathroom. The bath gets thrown out: there is to be a spacious shower instead. And the lavatory is going to have a fountain, like a bidet, and a blow dryer! One just presses a button when necessary, so to speak.

I wonder how long I will be able to press a button.

For a couple of days we are without a loo on the upper floor. It is rather tricky since the stair lift has not arrived and I can't use the stairs on my own. Mimmi buys the chemist's little Pimpinella potty. We test it with water but it's too heavy and I can't keep my balance. Ingrid suggests I simply sit on a nappy on the bed, then put it into a bag.

Good idea, but I'm afraid of leakage and put the nappy on a chair when I need it. Because my nerves and muscles are not co-ordinated my balance is hopeless – especially in the middle of the night. I fall off the chair, crashing into a floor vase with seven red roses in it from Olle.

Straight down on to the vase with a bare bottom.

It cracks and sort of bursts. Hisses.

'Olle, Olle, I'm sitting on splinters of glass,' I shout, or so I imagine. But my tongue is partially paralysed and not much is working in my throat.

Olle sleeps on.

It sounds like a roar from far away, but it's me.

If I move, the glass will cut me even more deeply.

'Olle!'

My husband always sleeps with ear-plugs and blindfold, which is the case tonight too.

At last:

'What's happened?'

'I fell over!'

He picks me up and, in the dark, he just makes out the blood.

'Have you got your period?'

'No, I'm bleeding. It's glass!' I whimper.

Now the surgeon takes over.

'Lie on your stomach,' he says.

Reluctantly I expose my backside.

'Damn! This needs stitches!'

I cry.

He brings out compresses, distilled water, tweezers, a needle, suture thread and a hypodermic with local anaesthetic.

From the wardrobe.

He picks pieces of glass out of my buttocks and has to stitch and fix me in three places. The situation is so bizarre that I can't stop myself laughing.

Laughter is a release.

Laughter keeps away the pain.

Black humour has saved many.

When he has put me to bed he arranges two roses in a

glass vase. Five were crushed by my fall. Despite every-thing, roses are still roses.

By the way, that ramp at the front works excellently for the wheelchair.

But it's used mostly for the boys' bicycles and toy cars.
It might turn into a mini golf-course too.

Gustaf's gym shorts, thinly encrusted with frost, are hanging on the balcony to air.

Soon the rowanberries will lose their bitterness and fatten the bullfinches and waxwings. The funnel chanterelles survive the frost and I miss wandering beneath the fir trees.

In the forest, where the smells are intense, the light filtered and the moss damp, I have dreamt of laying myself down to die.

No weariness of life, no longing for death, just a profound closeness to and unquestionable affinity with nature.

It was in the forest, by a lake, that I acquired my second skin: Mimmi.

When we shared her liver-pâté sandwiches with thin slices of pickled cucumber, and our three sons played at the edge of the trees, we didn't know that she would rub ointment on my bottom against bedsores.

When we exchanged secrets on the warm flat rocks and

became friends 'halfway through my life', as I then believed, we didn't know that she would lay her hand on my forehead and say, 'I shall never leave you. I'll be with you all the way to the end, and then I'll take care of your daughters and your sons.'

This is exactly what I need: touch, comfort and to feel trust.

A maxim coined by Hippocrates, the father of medicine, instructs:

'Seldom cure, often ease, always comfort.'

The medical profession today often cures, often eases, but what about comfort?

How can it find time for the comfort aspect of care?

I meet many comforters, among those whom doctors call 'auxiliaries'. Home care: Olga from St Petersburg, Aden from Somalia, Inger from Viggbyholm, Lisa from Täby, Inez from Lithuania.

I meet them before the council and the social-security office have finished investigating me and decided that I am subject to 'LSS according to paragraph 9:2 and paragraph 1:3'. This is the Law on Support and Service to people with functional disorders.

Lindquist has a permanent functional disorder, which leads to difficulties in her daily way of life and a comprehensive need for help, with personal hygiene, visits to the toilet, dressing and undressing, help at mealtimes and with communication . . . the functional disorder clearly does not depend upon natural ageing.

So, thanks to that, I now have my comforters.

Mimmi has been employed, and Ingrid, who is a professional.

I am the third woman with this diagnosis whom she has cared for until the end.

She says she will not leave me.

Her last patient, Ragna, died peacefully in her sleep.

Ragna had such difficulty with swallowing that she was given a tube in her stomach.

'She often wanted red wine so then I injected it into her stomach.'

'But she wouldn't have been able to taste it,' I object.

'I soaked a compress in wine and let her suck it,' replies Ingrid, and continues, 'When she wanted cheese, I made a bag and put some pieces into it so she could suck that too. Ragna loved Grevé cheese.'

One day when Gustaf arrives home and Ingrid is pottering in the kitchen, he studies her from head to toe, then asks, 'What job do you do really?'

'This is my job.'

'So what do you do?'

'I look after your mummy.'

'How long are you going to do that?'

'As long as she needs me.'

Many of the people I have spoken to in the medical profession believe that there are more ALS patients now than there were fifteen or twenty years ago. But there is no scientific evidence that the illness is becoming more common. At the same time, the technique for diagnosing ALS has improved. In the past patients languished in geriatric wards without a diagnosis.

But although diagnosis is easier, the cause of this incurable disease is unknown.

Why?

When I hoover the Internet for information I am surprised that so little research is being done on ALS. At the internationally renowned Karolinska Institute nobody is trying to solve the riddle of amyotrophic lateral sclerosis.

'Use me,' I suggest to the neurologist, but nobody has been in touch.

It clearly doesn't happen like that.

But why no research on ALS?

Martin Ingvar, professor and researcher on the brain, answers: 'It is difficult to conduct research on such an uncommon illness as ALS. There is no single reason why people are struck down. That makes it hard to get research going. Large-scale co-ordination is needed at an international level to get together big enough groups of patients. And the financing of research is split, which doesn't help this type of work.'

'More people suffer from brain-related diseases than from cancer. Why is so much more research being carried out on cancer?' I ask.

'Half of all the funds that we in the west use on medical diagnosis and care go to disorders of the nervous system. Yet it's true that only five per cent of research funding goes to this sector. Cancer research has been more successful in demonstrating that a cure is within reach and in improving palliative treatment – that research is important in the treatment of patients. We neuroscientists should publicize our successes. Those who fund research must be told that it's good business to invest more in neuro-research.'

'Is it possible to repair injured nerves by transplanting stem cells?'

'There is talk all the time about stem cells in connection with illnesses that are hard to cure. Motor-neurones will be particularly hard to replace with transplanted cells, since they are so long. On the other hand I think that research on stem cells will contribute knowledge about which cell-biological factors play a part in making a motor-neurone develop or atrophy. It is only when one knows the causes that one can find a more effective treatment.'

'And the causes of ALS are still unclear. Do you believe that any good treatment will be available in the future?'

'The finding of a cure for ALS lies in a better understanding of the biological mechanisms that lie behind the loss of motor-neurones. It can only be won through basic research conducted over the long term.'

The French Dining Room at the Grand Hôtel in Stockholm has existed since the hotel opened in 1874, and its culinary standards are high. It's been ages since we ate such exquisite food.

We are having a family celebration. If your time is limited, every celebration becomes the greatest.

I am wearing a dark red, draped velvet dress and we are sitting at a round table. The waiter moves it closer to the wall so that I can rest my head against the wooden panelling.

I ask to exchange the long-stemmed wine-glass for a tumbler and bend forward to sip the wine through a black straw.

Here we sit in velvet on red tapestry upholstery beneath cut-glass chandeliers, and Olle carefully lifts a piece of suckling pig to my lips. The meat melts in my mouth and the seasoning is full of surprises – caraway, thyme and aniseed, with the northern Swedish cheese in the potato gratin.

The French couple at the neighbouring table stare boldly in an unFrench way when Olle dries my lips with a linen table napkin. However, the lady at a table a little further away smiles encouragingly. I smile back and know that she is a soulmate. She and her companion use sign language.

So many words are used to fill emptiness. Words are putty to fill cracks. To keep the darkness away and the lies alive.

When we believe that everything has been said, the most important thing is left. The thing we defend ourselves against.

When there are no more words, only the truth remains.

Here we sit and converse with only a few words.

I am closer to my husband than ever before.

Closer to myself.

When he has wiped the blackberry soufflé from my chin, we take the taxi service for the disabled home.

The Swedish ladies' football team is about to win the silver medal in the World Championships. We lie on the bed, the boys, Olle and I, watching the match and eating oat-milk ice-cream. I get a lot of mucus if I have cow's milk, and it's difficult to cough it up nowadays.

Pontus often lies behind me as though we were two spoons in a drawer.

'They ought to play more defensively,' he yells in my ear.

'Mummy, can you play as well as that?' asks Gustaf in the break.

'I can't play at all, you nutcase.'

'Last summer you shot and even headed a ball.'

'Did I?'

'How are you, by the way?'

'I'm fine. Although I'm ill.'

'Yes, I know that, and we're not going to talk about it. You know – I said.'

'OK. But my feet are freezing. You can have five kronor if you massage them.'

And he does. I can see that he likes it. It's good, because then he's sharing in it all. He, the little one, doesn't want to talk, but to touch his sick mother and make her comfortable, that must feel good.

'Fetch my purse so that I can give you the money.'

'No, Mummy, you keep it.'

Before they go to bed Pontus thinks about a new language. Blinks may become complicated. We could learn the tap language of prisoners, but that might be too difficult.

'We can write different things you want to do on bits of paper. Every paper will have a number and you blink that many times.'

'But three blinks will still work?'

This morning they are eating yoghurt and muesli. I can tell this from the sound.

It will be a relief when the stair lift arrives. Then perhaps I can sit with them while they eat. As I did before. Two months ago.

'Take a piece of paprika and an apple. Do you want yoghurt or porridge?'

At present they eat alone. They choose their own clothes. They come upstairs to me and hug me: 'Bye-bye and have a good day, Mummy.'

'Ha'e you bwushed your teesh?'

They always have.

Today my carer and I make the trip to physiotherapy at Huddinge Hospital. I am given the ventilator I've heard so much about.

I don't like it.

It fires off a strong puff into the lungs, then I have to blow it out.

In this way the poisonous carbon dioxide that remains in the lungs when you breathe as I do is cleared out.

I feel like a balloon.

Puff!

It's like when you stick your head out of a train window.

I'm scared of the mask.

If I pretend it's a headwind at sea, perhaps I can distract myself.

Or I shall have to turn myself into a beetle.

'What are you going to do with it when I don't need it any more?'

'You can return it to us.'

'Well, it won't be me, exactly.'

'No, oh dear, sorry!'

So it's going to be used again. Good.

The ventilator costs the taxpayers thirty thousand kronor.

I cost the community quite a lot.

In two weeks' time, the turbo-wheelchair worth a hundred thousand kronor is due to arrive. The stair lift costs sixty thousand.

A computer operated by your nose: twenty thousand. It should arrive the day after tomorrow. Lucky, because now I write mostly with just my middle finger. A page-turner: twenty thousand. Disability adaptation of the home: at least eighty thousand kronor.

Gustaf thinks all this is cool: 'It's so fantastic, Mummy. A wheelchair with blinkers, the meanest wickedest keyboard, the meanest wickedest parking card, the meanest wickedest everything. You get them all for nothing, and you're not even working. Look at Daddy. He has to pay for everything.'

I'm starting to feel more and more like one of the patients on ward nineteen at the Vasa Hospital in Gothenburg in 1975. Now the old hospital in Aschebergsgatan is an attractive part of the Chalmers University of Technology. Then it was a geriatric hospital, the terror of the citizens of Gothenburg. It was a terminus in the full meaning of the word.

I had often met death before: horses, people and dogs.

But this was different.

'You can come with me to Klara. She's in the last stage now, lying in the linen storeroom.'

Eva Gustafsson is an assistant nurse. She lives on Hisingen. After she and I have washed and wrapped a few bodies in shrouds during a shift we become friends.

Later on I will leave a five-thousand kronor deposit with a landlord in Västra Frölunda for a two-room flat in Hisingsgatan.

But for now I rent a room in the nurses' home. There, the gulls steal my breakfast, because we have to hang food in a plastic carrier-bag outside on the hasp of the window. There is no fridge.

As we change Klara's drawsheet, she dies. Like a feeble gasp. A sigh.

Eva shows me how to take care of a dead person.

When the relatives arrive, Klara is lying in clean sheets. She has her false teeth in, her hair is combed, her night-dress clean, her jaw bound up, her hands clasped, a candle is burning, and she is lying – for the first time in the geriatric ward – in a single room.

I stay on ward nineteen for five months, take care of many like Klara and receive the training required to qualify as a physiotherapist.

It is Mrs Mattsson who causes me to change direction and start asking questions.

'What is dignity?'

'Integrity?'

'Human dignity?'

Mrs Mattsson is, perhaps, sixty and has severe diabetes. Her toes have blackened and rotted, since her blood circulation is poor. We cut off bits of toe, as we are supposed to.

Mrs Mattsson is blind. Her mind is completely clear.

One day both her legs are amputated. Without her knowledge. She lies in bed and waves the stumps. She tries to reach her feet with her hands. Feet that are no longer there. And her blind eyes are crying.

At that point I applied to the College of Journalism, passed the tests and was the youngest on the course.

I was convinced that I and no one else would reveal the truth.

'If I am here when you die,' says Ingrid, 'and if the children come home from school, what do you want me to do?'

'What do you mean?' I ask, and try to ward off fear.

'I mean if I haven't had time to get you in order.'

Klara in ward nineteen flashes through my mind.

'Then they can help you comb my hair and so on.'

'Good. I agree with that. It would be so difficult to head them off.'

'But I won't die just like that? You should be able to tell beforehand?'

She doesn't reply, but fiddles with a flannel.

I don't ask again.

She turns me on my side and props me up with a pillow at my back.

'Will you dress me,' I say, in a small voice, 'in pyjamas?'

As though I'm wondering which clothes are prescribed.

'You can wear your tracksuit or whatever you like.'

I don't want to talk any more.

It's weird to live in a sick body.

Mimmi struggles out of her threadbare jeans and tight T-shirt and strides over to me. I'm sitting naked in a shower-chair. She has on tiny black string panties and a matching lacy bra.

'Today, my Pulla, you're going to have the full hair-conditioning treatment.'

She calls me that because it rhymes with Ulla. Her humour is often below the belt and she is good at rhyming.

I love water. I love feeling the warmth run down over my body and I love it when she leans my head against her breasts. I burrow into her deep cleavage, trusting.

Later, at the computer, I want to say something, but it's too hard. I write instead:

'Mimmi, I'm becoming more and more dependent on you.

I can't do without you.'

She writes her answer: 'And I can't do without you. The fact is, I can't imagine what it will be like when you're no longer here.'

'Have you got the strength to help me? You've got to have a life of your own!'

'My Pulla, I have a life of my own where, just at the moment, you take up a lot of space. I shan't fail you. I have the strength and I shall be with you all the time.'

'You helped look after your mother when she was ill, and now you have me. Where do you get your strength from?'

'I don't know, but I've learnt from my two older sisters. We're alike. They've always been my examples, always there for me when I've needed them.'

'Do you think one can feel joy in giving help and comfort?'

'I'm convinced of it. Not to be there at times of hardship would make me suffer even more.'

Then no more words come to me.

Would I have given her so much time if she had been ill?

We look at each other and there is a sudden twinkle in our eyes. We break out of our serious mood.

'Are you going to brush my teeth now or what?'

'I was wondering if you'd ever ask me that! Your breath's been stinging my nostrils for quite a while now,' she replies.

The thin-as-gauze veil between tragic and comic.

The laughter that disarms.

'Mimmi, what will you do if I die when you're here? Just like that.'

'I don't know.'

'You must tie an elastic bandage round my head so that when my body stiffens my mouth isn't stuck open. And I want my hands crossed on my breast. Not clasped. I want to have pink linen pyjamas and the dried lavender that's lying over there by the TV.'

'Why the lavender?'

'It's mine. I sowed it by the south wall in Skåne.'

'I shall wash you and make you look pretty and light a candle.'

'Yes, OK,' I reply impatiently. 'Don't be afraid if I breathe out when you turn me over.'

'How do you know about that?'

'I prepared thirteen corpses on ward nineteen.'

'I'll cope.'

'Tell the children I'll feel cold when they touch me. And we must buy the elastic bandage.'

'You're such a control freak!'

'You've changed,' says my friend from work. 'You don't accept any beating about the bush. It's just straight to the point nowadays.'

Yes, that's right. So much has been peeled away.

The thick fog that previously obscured the view has lifted.

I have taken my place in the look-out tower and observe myself from a distance.

My self-esteem is strong. My self-confidence has recovered, almost.

In my experience, the intellect becomes keener at the same rate as the body declines.

What have I spent my time on in the past?

I draw on the threads of my memory. I now spend perhaps fourteen of every twenty-four hours in bed. When the bustle has settled, in my imagination I row the little boat out to the middle of the bay. The dog sits in the bow and her damp brown nose quivers as she sniffs in the direction of the mainland to the east.

My oar strokes are strong and I am enjoying the sight

of the blades cutting through the water. It swirls, and the wash makes me happy. I have a landmark, so the line from the stern is straight.

These are my home waters and it's before the age of compulsory life-jackets. It is an honour to burn my young freckled skin until it blisters and is cooled with potato flour in the light of the paraffin lamp. Times have changed.

To the west of the channel, where the cargo boats carry timber and coke, I lift the oars from the rowlocks, lie down and let the south-westerly carry me home without oars. The cotton-wool clouds in the sky are moving faster than the wind down here on Lake Vänern. A light breeze is blowing and an occasional mewing is the only sound the seagulls make.

Every summer I drift without oars. Ingemar Johansson becomes world champion. Dag Hammarskjöld and John F. Kennedy die. Krushchev shows his anger in the UN by banging with his shoe. I cry over the dog Laika, and can sing the whole of 'Kalinka' with Monica Zetterlund. I know how one lays to at a jetty and I can tie hitches and knots.

I have a mother and father.

Who will powder my sons' burnt shoulders with potato flour?

Who will warm the grey stone in the iron stove and wrap it in a towel to warm cold feet?

Who will blow out their paraffin lamp?

When one drifts without oars it is important to lift them out of the rowlocks.

How does a middle-aged person who has always praised independence and autonomy learn to accept being cared for like a child?

How does a woman who still wants to be attractive to her husband learn to accept that in all probability she no longer is?

'I'm ready!' I shout from the loo.

He lifts me up, flushes, and tries to haul me in the direction of the bedroom.

'No,' I wail. 'No!'

'What do you want?'

He does not understand my reply, 'trousers'. It sounds like a slurred 'trou'ash'.

I struggle when he tries to lead me forwards.

'Darling, what is it?'

'Trou'ash!' Now I beat the arm I can still move against my legs, and weeping overwhelms me.

At last my husband sees that my pyjama trousers are round my ankles and that my backside is bare. I bend, knock-kneed, as if to hide myself, when he reaches down to pull them up.

'But that wasn't so bad,' he protests, when I sob loudly.

No, perhaps it wasn't, but now, just at this moment, it *is* that bad.

It's the powerlessness. It gushes up, and is only getting worse.

'I feel as though I shall perhaps be dead by Christmas,' I hear myself say when we have gone to bed. (Attention-seeking?)

'Really?' (He doesn't protest.)

'Don't know.'

More crying.

'Poor little one!' (Surely it's not only me who should be pitied?)

'We have to discuss where you stand on the issue of hospital care,' he continues.

'You talk as though I'm going to die now,' I hit out.

'It was you who said that about Christmas. You must understand that you might have to stay in hospital towards the end.'

'Never a geriatric ward,' I howl. (Klara, ward nineteen, Mrs Mattsson and the smell of corpse.)

'Are you afraid of dying?'

Shake my head.

'Is it the children?'

Shake my head.

'We have to consider the children. It mustn't alarm

them.'

'It's normal to die,' I whimper, in the foetal position, my back to him.

'It's hard to be terminally ill. Hard to accept.'

'What the hell do you know about it? Have you read it in a medical book or what?'

'But, darling,' he says gently, 'the Stockholm nursing home is very nice and they accept ALS patients.'

'You've already checked,' I snap.

The weeping will not stop. I dribble and snivel.

'Darling, you know you want us to talk openly and you would have checked if I were as ill as you.' (Correct!) 'Are you so afraid of dying?'

'No, I'm afraid of being alone. I'm afraid of being deserted.'

Now I allow myself to be comforted and fall asleep against his shoulder after he promises that only death will separate us.

I will be able to die at home 'if that's possible' and he will be with me to the end.

'You must be my husband, not my doctor. I must be able to trust you,' I say, in a small voice, and he replies that I can.

'Mummy, today I cried when we were playing football in the school playground.'

He is sitting beside me on the bed and his dark blue eyes are ponds, filled to the brim.

'My teacher came and asked what was wrong.'

'What did you say?'

'That you're ill.'

'But she knew that, didn't she?'

'Not everything. Not how ill you are.'

'What happened?'

'She started to cry too.'

'Would you like Daddy or your teacher to tell the whole class? That might make it easier for you.'

'I don't know.'

I don't either. Will he be bullied? Treated in a special way? Over-protected?

I send an email to Ken Chesterton on the children's trauma team at Vrinnevi Hospital in Norrköping. I receive a reply immediately:

It is good if the teacher knows how things are with you, and that your boy knows that his teacher knows. If he knows that his teacher understands how things might be for him, it will mean a great deal to him. Some teachers know more, others less, about how children may react to difficult events/information. We usually inform teachers of common reactions to be certain of increased tolerance towards the children concerned. Common reactions are, apart from the upset that your boy shows, difficulty in concentrating, difficulty in remembering, and tiredness. Anger is also common, especially among boys.

Re info to the class. Ask your boy if he wants the class to know, and if he does, whether he wants to be present when the class is told or if he wants to arrive after the teacher has told them. The discussion above naturally concerns both boys, even if the eldest shows his sadness more openly at the moment.

Gustaf still doesn't want to hear about the illness. He is angry because I speak so badly.

'Talk so that I understand,' he says, and looks at me as though he doesn't recognize me.

I ask him to hold the mask when I have to breathe using it.

Then he comes close.

We have to get a grip on this.

Olle and I call a meeting.

Early one morning we sit at the dining-table, drink coffee and eat Italian almond biscuits.

Gustaf's teacher, Pontus's teacher, the school nurse, Olle and I.

The atmosphere is a little tense.

I hear Olle tell them about me.

'It's difficult for everyone, naturally, not least for the boys.'

The teachers nod and nibble the biscuits.

I am in a void. It feels unreal to be sitting here.

I look around me and see the flowers I have been given.

The picture we bought when we got engaged.

'. . . an illness that progresses very fast . . .'

The copper barrel that came from my great-grandmother Hanna's kitchen.

'. . . strikes down a hundred and fifty Swedes each year . . .'

The fabric samples for the curtains that I still have not chosen.

'. . . isn't infectious and she has not caused it . . .'

The photo of when I caught a pike weighing five kilos.

'. . . can't walk on her own any longer . . .'

Photos of the boys and me in the forest.

My gaze lingers there and the mask cracks.

The teachers start to cry too and the school nurse brings out the tissues.

'I knew it would be like this so I didn't put on any mascara,' snivels one.

'Mine's waterproof,' says the other.

When we've all wiped our noses, it turns into a good meeting.

The school nurse is going to get in touch with the vicar and the psychologist, and the children's friends might also need support.

Pontus's teacher tells us that he said, 'My mummy is going to die,' the day she found him crying in the playground during a ballgame.

The school nurse says it's good that he 'can verbalize it'. That he has insight.

Gustaf is probably the one who needs most help. He is happier and brighter than usual.

'Some cry, but it's just as common for them not to.'

One can feel numb.

Everyone reacts differently.

'You've become so frail and fragile, yet you're strong,' says my younger daughter Carin gently, and creeps up close. 'When I hold you you're so delicate and tiny. Before, you were physically so strong, but weak. You were a seeker and wanted to please everyone. You rushed back and forth and were never satisfied. All I wanted was to have a day with you alone, but I never did. You never had time.'

'Didn't I?'

'No. Now you've stopped seeking. Now, when you're ill, you've found yourself. And now you have peace.'

I want to defend myself against that thing about time. But I realize that would be wrong: her truth is hers alone.

'Can you learn anything from this?' I say.

'To be satisfied with what I have. Not to postpone things. That life is fragile.'

Carin celebrates her twenty-first birthday with us.

She is given a special cake, and she points out discreetly that it is her elder sister's favourite, not hers.

'Oh dear.'

I'm sitting in the wheelchair beside her bed and grief stabs me when I remember that this is the last time I will celebrate her birthday. She's clearly thinking the same thing.

Just at that moment our eyes do not meet.

My younger daughter Carin is not an ordinary person. She is not only made of flesh and blood.

'I'm made of flesh, blood and potato,' she used to say, when she was little and was in her 'thoughtsies'.

I am sitting in a wheelchair by her bed, and the day of her birth twenty-one years ago is vivid in black and white.

'Your baby is malformed. She is in an incubator and you can see her later.'

My child has a tumour where her bottom should be, a tumour larger than her head. It is dark blue and I dare not touch it during the minute I am allowed to hold her.

I think I can probably make a pair of trousers with braces and space for the tumour, but how will we manage the nappies?

My newborn baby is quiet and beautiful, and the corners of her mouth turn up.

'It must be better to have too much on one's body than not enough,' says her father.

And that's true.

She has an operation, but there is still too much of her, and that has to be cut away, too, over the years.

I remember that my Grandma always searched for four-leafed clovers in the late spring, and they are also a kind of malformation.

When the virus took up residence in Carin's brain, when the king was on his traditional visit to eastern Sweden, I brooded about what the point of it all was.

She was almost two and had stopped walking and seeing light, and we had to start again from the beginning.

And we have succeeded, although there have been a number of painful skids off the road.

I force away the sadness and try to be happy when she sits by my bed tonight and whispers the secrets of a twenty-one-year-old into my ear. The moon is waning. It releases its light over the water and all the way into the room and my daughter's forehead.

The planet Mars continues to stare with its skin-diver's mask, slightly paler now as it and Earth move away from each other. For this time round.

There is a life cycle in space too.

Growing up with twenty-three apple trees, two plum trees, a pear tree and several dozen metres of berry bushes in rows allows for plenty of escape routes and hiding-places.

And living a stone's throw from Granny, with Schubert and a Steinway grand, and two throws from Grandma, with apron and plain buns, offers me refuge, like a fawn in flight.

And that is often necessary.

When Daddy descends into darkness.

He makes his bed in the darkness and is unreachable.

'I bring up my children and dogs in the same way.'

The dogs are firmly drilled. They cringe.

I put my yoghurt bowl down beside the dogs' bowls and lick it up on all fours.

Can you see me now?

Grandma and Granny are my safe zones. Their love is unconditional.

'Come here, dear heart, and look at this orchid. Look

at the stamen and the pistil. Such symmetry. You must understand that there is a creator's hand behind all this. That God exists.'

In the summers I sometimes stay at Granny and Grandad's summer house with one of my cousins. There are about twenty of us. We are given ginger biscuits, and milk in brown bottles. From the towers of the dilapidated old mansion we watch the cargo ships that breathe of foreign shores.

When a boat with a red stripe and an A turns up, it makes Granny happy: she has shares in Ahlmark's.

Grandad is a dentist and so is Mummy. She works hard to support us all, and her white clogs make drum rolls on the parquet.

We stand to attention at the dinner-table, my big brother and I, and chew our roast reindeer quietly when at last Daddy has given us permission to sit.

I learn discipline, self-control and self-restraint.

Characteristics that are both bad and good.

And I get a great deal of fresh air and nourishing food.

We discuss it, my brother and I, one afternoon when he has taken the day off from his job in Karlstad to visit me.

Receiving visits is a true benefit of illness. The doctors speak of a 'secondary benefit of illness'. I wonder what the primary one is. The illness itself?

We talk about the past, my brother and I, and remember how we used to hide in Hanna's copper barrel.

Now it is here in my home. We nibble rocket salad, sheep's cheese and sun-dried tomatoes and I say it was lucky we didn't suffocate in it. Nowadays children do die when they're playing and shut each other in. But we never let the other stay in the barrel longer than he or she wanted.

My brother tells me about the cancer that has been removed from his lungs and how it has changed him.

He has reverted to being as he used to be, I think, before he was weighed down and bound up.

He is much happier now.

And so am I.

Now he's had a cancer operation and the scar's red, and I have my thing, we're both happier.

'Where does the strength come from,' he wonders.

'It's inside us, but we haven't needed it before. The buzz of life has been too loud,' I reply.

Self-control is probably quite a good thing too.

We chat about the hut, the blockhouse, which Daddy built and for which Mummy made the flag.

We laugh at the military discipline: the Swedish flag had to be lowered 'at sundown or at the latest at nine o'clock'.

We stood to attention, naturally, and I dare not think what would have happened if we had dropped the flag on the ground.

Two blond, straight-backed children.

My brother thinks I exaggerate.

My truth is mine alone.

When evening comes I ask him to pull me up a little further in bed.

He lifts all of me and I laugh with joy.

A year ago today, following the terrorist attack on Bali, I interviewed an expert from the Consumers' Insurance Office about the fact that young people often do not bother with insurance when they travel. It was raining, I remember. The photographer wanted me to carry the tripod and I did, despite the slipped disc in my neck – thought then to be the cause of the problems with my hand. That was what I hoped at any rate.

Camera tripods are heavy, and the fact that I could carry it seems odd to me now.

Now I can't even lift a fork to my mouth, let alone a glass. I can't scratch my forehead and—it's pointless to list all the things I cannot do.

In the course of a year I have become a prisoner in my body.

A year ago I carried a tripod along Sveavägen in Stockholm.

Today I am fed strained food.

A year ago I asked questions about travel insurance.

Today I'm checking over my life insurance.

But.

I can laugh.

Hug my four children, or at least lift my left arm so that I can touch them.

Hug my husband, and kiss him with my semi-paralysed mouth.

Read.

Listen to music.

Breathe fresh air.

Wander in the labyrinth of my memory.

Listen to friends.

Peace . . . ?

Feel peace within me!

(Sometimes.)

The reception area for Neurology at the Karolinska Hospital is run-down and gloomy. It looks dreadful. The patients' lavatory is often dirty and stinks of urine.

It's a pity. As a patient, it affects me: the environment depresses me, makes me feel less valuable.

Must visit the Radiology Home and see how things are for those who have cancer.

I am sitting here now, in the reception area at Neurology, watching. As usual, I observe and ponder.

I see a shabby man with stained trousers and spasms. Parkinson's, perhaps. A young woman in a wheelchair. MS? Another man who seems healthy. Or is he doing as I am and hiding his diseased body part?

I hide my useless hand in a pashmina shawl.

And then the door opens and a man enters. No, he doesn't 'enter', he glides in.

Like a St Lucia.

With a straight back.

In a dignified manner.

Slowly.

His head rests on what looks like a cake dish with a stand and he wears a crown of thorns.

He sits down opposite me.

And smiles.

The man with the crown of thorns meets my eyes and his are as clear as glass, and blue.

'Hallo,' I say.

'Hallo!'

'May I . . .'

'Yes, you may.'

'. . . ask . . . why you have that . . . thing . . . frame . . . on your head?'

'I have broken my neck.'

'In that case you should be dead!'

'Not necessarily. I'm alive.'

'Would you like to explain to me?'

He likes me asking questions.

'Most people get scared and look away.'

The light metal frame he has on his head keeps it still. It's a 'halo-jacket'. Sometimes the step from halo to crown of thorns is short.

'What happened?'

'It was early one morning. I was going birdwatching. Binoculars dangling on my chest and a Thermos of coffee in my rucksack. The sun was shining and I cycled on the road by Järva Field. It was only five and I thought I was alone with the birds. I came to a crossroads, and after that . . .'

'What happened?'

'Along came a car with a man who also thought he had the road to himself. But, of course, I was there. So we collided.'

'Do you remember anything?'

'Yes indeed. I remember that my fingers ploughed through the gravel. I can still hear the sound of stones rolling.'

'You remember it that vividly?'

'Yes, I can feel the gravel scratching my hand.'

We are interrupted. It is my turn.

Autumn comes and the vicar cycles to my home on her mountain bike.

She has picked a rose.

I don't get any answers to my questions, for although she is ordained she has doubts.

She reads from the Book of Job and tells me of how he curses God:

'God has wronged me and drawn his net around me /. . ./ He has blocked my way so that I cannot pass; he has shrouded my paths in darkness /. . ./ He tears me down on every side till I am gone,' says Job (19:6–10).

The Lord blesses Job anyway with fourteen thousand sheep, six thousand camels, a thousand pairs of oxen and a thousand female donkeys. He lived until he was a hundred and forty and died 'old and full of years'.

The vicar tells me this to help me understand that it's OK to doubt and be angry.

I turn to the sea and find my peace.

'Hi, Mum. Are you alive or not?'

'Hi. I'm alive.'

'Good.'

'How is the eczema on your hand?'

'It itches. Why do I get eczema?'

'It can be the result of worry and stress.'

'Stress is really stupid. Like being angry or upset or emotional.'

'Do you think so? Stress is stupid, but I think it's fine to be emotional. You must remember how I cried when I watched *The Lion King*.'

'A grown-up who cries because of a cartoon is really—'

'Are you worried, Gustaf?'

'Because you're ill?'

'Yes.'

'Sometimes. Not when I play football. You can't run around and think at the same time.'

'No, clearly not.'

'No.'

'In a week's time I'm going into hospital to have a tube in my tummy.'

'What sort of tube?'

'To have soup through.'

'Why?'

'Such a lot gets stuck in my throat. With the tube the food will go straight into my tummy.'

'But are you going to have a tube that just hangs out?'

'I think it's short and can be connected to a longer one.'

'God, that's really wicked!'

'I was sad last night, Mummy.'

'Tell me, Pontus.'

'You're just getting sicker.'

'Yes, I know.'

'And you're going to die.'

'Everyone does.'

'But I don't know anyone who has a dead mother.'

'They rang from the hospital,' says my carer, 'and you're going to get a hole in your stomach as early as Tuesday. I spoke to your doctor too.'

'On Tuesday! It was supposed to be in a week's time.'

'They think they should bring it forward. You only weigh forty-nine kilos now.'

'Why didn't they want to speak to me? Why didn't they tell me?'

'They thought I could.'

'Bloody hell, no!'

This was wrong of the doctors. I might be terminally ill and unable to express myself comprehensibly, but I have no problem in understanding.

The doctor should have informed me, not my carer.

It should be obvious.

I'm furious.

'They also said that you will have to stay in the neuro-logical ward for three days.'

'Stay there! No way! It's Gustaf's ninth birthday then.'

'Yes, well, they said you have to stay there. It's important that the tube is adjusted correctly.'

'I refuse.'

'But, Ulla-Carin, it's for your own sake. And I'll come and visit you.'

'No. No visitors.'

'But—'

'I'll have to be in hospital for Gustaf's birthday and I'll never come home again.'

Sobs tear me to pieces and wear me out. I'm aching with sadness and fury. And I'm outraged by their having talked over my head.

'I'm going to end up in a geriatric ward.'

She lays my damp head in her lap. But that doesn't defuse the anger.

The situation is not improved by Mimmi and Olle telling me how worn out they are, that they never get to sleep through the night.

I am becoming a burden.

That's how it is.

They deny this.

Naturally, they deny that I am a burden.

I am told that I give orders.

'Water!'

'Medicine!'

'The loo!'

True, I have to save words. Can only manage a few.

Have to breathe. My voice has lost all shades of intonation. It's a monotonous croak.

I hate this new voice.

Will try to sound more friendly. Sure.

The day disappears in emotional outbursts.

I can only meet the children's eyes.

No Kafka and beetle to help me.

Not even Imre Kertész and Köves are at hand.

Today I sink a little more and become a slightly different person.

Less capable.

It doesn't even help when Olle whispers, 'I promised to love you for better or for worse.'

I turn away my head.

To self-elected loneliness.

The maple leaves glow red against the frostbitten country-side. A little snow lies in the blueberry brush and the boys are tobogganing on the bare rocky slab.

Winter is here and we're going to carve faces in pump-kins and put them to light up our front steps.

In Canada they celebrated Hallowe'en with deadly seriousness. One of our neighbours had skeletons and gravestones made of painted Styrofoam in the garden. He used to put something out on the steps to attract cats, and they crowded there in the evenings.

One evening, with lots of children and lots of sweets, Gustaf disappeared. Hordes of them ran between the houses and begged for 'treats'. But not my seven-year-old.

It was raining and the darkness was impenetrable.

I rushed from house to house.

'Have you seen a little boy dressed up as a ghost?'

There were hundreds of them. All the seven-year-old boys were wearing skeleton costumes.

At last I saw a well-known silhouette. Leaning for-wards. Energetic. Soaked to the skin.

'Mummy, why are you crying?'

'I'm so happy to see you.'

'Do you want some sweets?'

For dinner we had pumpkin soup in pumpkin bowls laid on maple leaves, and it was among the most delicious and beautiful meals I had ever eaten.

To cook and eat food is pleasurable.

This evening I'm eating my last real meal. Not a meal like I had when I was healthy, but a meal as they are now.

Chopped and mashed crab topped with a little lobster sauce and crumbled tarragon.

Cut-up baby spinach warmed in lemon oil, the stalks removed.

Avocado mousse.

Half a glass of white wine.

Mimmi feeds me carefully. I drink the wine through a straw in tiny – not sips, something much smaller.

After this, fasting.

Early tomorrow morning I'm going to hospital and there I will be given the hole for tube-feeding.

In the morning Gustaf comes in to celebrate a little of his birthday with me, and my mother-in-law lays the tray.

'It's probably good for the boys to see you in hospital,' says Olle, when I say despondently that I don't want any visitors.

It's the first time I'll be away from home because I'm ill.

I'm scared.

I'll think about meals I've enjoyed.

Tomorrow I'll think with happiness about food I've eaten.

The crab yesterday evening was delicious.

I notice again: to experience something for the last time can be more intense than it was the first.

The door is locked when we arrive at the neurology ward.

'One of our patients runs away all the time,' explains the nurse who lets us in.

I am given a single room, with a microphone and two cameras so that the staff can keep an eye on me.

'The epilepsy room. The cameras are so that we can keep a check in case a patient has a fit, but it's your room now. Have you brought your own clothes, by the way?'

'No. If I'm in hospital I should have hospital clothes.'

I am weighed. They inform us that I am suffering from dehydration and put me on a drip.

When Olle has left, I am gripped by fear and desolation. Will I ever go home again?

Wait for four hours and have mentally settled my accounts several times when the porter arrives with Sister Margaretha from the ALS team.

'What are all the cables on the ceiling for?' I try to ask, as they push my bed along the Neuroroute in the hospital's subterranean corridors. But there is no answer: it is impossible to understand the slurred speech as thick as porridge after the patient has had 'something to calm you'.

'It's like a local anaesthetic at the dentist's,' says the anaesthetist, and squirts liquid into my throat.

I'm suffocating!

Can't swallow!

Mucus wells up and here comes the doctor with a black tube, which he threads into my stomach via my anaesthetized gullet. The surgeon stands on my other side, and when her scalpel meets the black tube's lamp she makes her incision and puts into position the rubber tube that will provide me with nourishment from now on.

It's quick. I am so panic-stricken and faint that I'm given oxygen to bring me round.

I have been given an umbilical cord.

Like a newborn.

All nourishment reaches me through it.

I am now fed for eighteen hours a day.

'I'm here for you and you're here for me,' whispers Sister Karin. She holds my hand with both of hers and doesn't turn her eyes away. 'We're here together and you are strong.'

'No, I'm faint and weak.'

'Yes, but you are strong here.' She points at my head.

She becomes my lodestar now.

They are talking over my head about me.

'She ought to have a drawsheet when we turn her.'

'Can she walk by herself?'

I am a third person. A 'she'.

The funny thing is that I like it. They are looking after me and I can just let it happen. I have my own sphere, my space, where nobody can reach me.

No demands. Free for my own thoughts.

And Gretel, the seaman's daughter from Åland, sees what I need.

'Would you like a bath?'

'Can't, as you see.'

'Yes, you can, we'll bathe you.'

She and Michelyn from Angola lay me in a bed-bath and fill it.

As long as my thoughts are free, I am inviolable.

I can think freely and am therefore independent.

They can wash my body and I can let myself enjoy it instead of feeling shame.

To surrender myself naked into their hands frees me.

Nobody can reach my soul.

They can be my oars and row for me, and I can lie on the deck and gaze at the heavens.

When at last I wake out of the grogginess, I feel a growing impatience in that epilepsy room. I have settled my accounts with life so many times, lying in the foetal position in the bed, with its drawsheet and plastic protection, that now I want to get on with my life.

I ask for a chaplain.

She arrives at once and my hand is so weak that she has to push the record-button on the tape-recorder.

'Sometimes when terribly hard things happen to you, you can arrive at a turning-point in life, although you may not see it as such. And people whom you may not have counted on in the past can be the ones to step forward and give new love and help.

'It can mean unexpected intimacy. That can sometimes be a turning-point, a new opportunity, in the midst of all the difficulties. All these people who have understood, and who want to be close, perhaps they are the most important people. The ones who dare to come close, and share both pain and pleasure.'

'What is death?'

'I imagine it as being taken out of time, bodily time, and the physical dimension. And whatever we were, our personality or what we sometimes call the soul, goes to God and we leave our body here. It returns to the earth. It belongs to the earth. But it also gives rise to new life.'

'What happens when you die?'

'Death for me has two faces. As a hospital chaplain, I've seen that. One is grief, pain and fear. But sometimes, just at the juncture between life and death, something else happens.

'Something very beautiful.

'Peaceful.

'The pain stops.

'A presence – so powerful that I can hardly describe it – is there when death is near and when it releases you.

'And then I don't feel afraid.

On the contrary, I can feel an unbelievable peace. Sometimes almost joy. Precisely in the borderland between life and death.'

'But what's the point of my having to die and leave four children, two of them young?'

'I find it hard to answer that question. I find it hard to see any meaning in this.'

'I want life to be just. But in these situations I can't find any answers. I can't. And even I feel pain and despair.

'And I cry to God:

"I see no point in this.

But stay close to me.

Embrace me."

'I think about you. And I think about your family, your children, too. That whatever happens, you should not let go of your love for your children and your husband, and those who are close to you.

'Don't let go of yourself.'

I need to feel the existence of an inner strength.

My chaplain has black beady eyes, crew-cut grey hair and eyebrows like black caterpillars.

Her hands enclose my left hand and she places a wooden cross on my table.

'One of the lines goes from the earth to heaven. The other from person to person. In the middle of the cross is you.'

She speaks softly and comfortingly, in metaphors.

'Something good can come out of this, even if you can't see it now.'

I dare to say that it will be so.

'In a wider perspective something new may happen, or something new may develop in the lives of those who have been involved with you.

'Rather like a seed that has been planted in the earth. It has to be covered by earth, but out of this little seed new life will grow. It isn't visible in the seed, but it will grow up and become something incredibly beautiful. Thanks to you.'

'Have you got any more images?'

'The butterfly starts in the cocoon. Then one day the cocoon falls off and the beautiful butterfly flies free. It flies wherever it wants to, no longer confined by the cocoon. And that's how I think sometimes of a person's life. Sometimes we are so limited – by illness perhaps, but it can also be by our life. It sort of shuts us in. It's a little symbolic of how we live today. We get nowhere. We're prisoners in our own existence. But when we dare to affirm life as it really is, both the life we have now and also our eternity, then we are free.'

'Sum up what's happening to me.'

'Your life is more than it is at present. Your life is greater than this moment of illness. That's the first thing. There is much more to life than your illness. Ulla-Carin is much more than ALS, which sets limits for you.

'The second thing is that you have a history behind you, which is also greater than this present moment in your life. All the people you have met. All your children. I don't know much about you, but I know that a person is always greater than her illness. See beyond everything that limits you.

'It's painful to say farewell to people and all the positive things that have happened to you. It hurts. But it is vital that you do it.'

It must be the last wasp of the year that flies in through the balcony door, fat and slow, but this one has survived the first frost and the first snow.

The wasp and I.

Ingrid hits at it with a newspaper to kill it.

'No, let it out and it'll die in due course.'

It is early in the morning and the first meal of the day will soon be over. We have got off to a flying start here at home. It is hard for me to endure being tethered for hours at a time. The machine is now pumping in two hundred millilitres per hour. This means that breakfast has taken two and a half hours.

I'm going to be fed through the tube for seven and a half hours today.

If this had happened in the past, before they were able to put ingenious tubes into people's stomachs, I would have been dead by now. If it had happened before the days when the medical system worked as well as it does now for a relatively young person like me, I would have been one of many patients with bedsores and cut-off toes in a geriatric ward.

Instead I am lying in my bed at home and I can smell the gunpowder smoke from Gustaf's new cap-gun. He is sitting on Olle's bed and firing wildly around him, even at me.

'Your grandfather, who was an officer, said that one should never aim at people unless it was deadly serious, in war or in self-defence.'

'Was Grandad in the war?'

'No, Sweden wasn't at war. But if we had been, Grandad would have taken part in it.'

'When you were in hospital, I earned some money.'

'How?'

'I cut the fingers off the gloves that Ingrid uses when she nurses you, and I sold them as condoms.'

'So that's why the box is empty!'

'Exactly.'

'Shall we watch my new film?' he wonders. He has just turned nine, and he lays down his weapon on the white duvet.

He holds my hand as we are absorbed in orcs', elves' and hobbits' lives for two hours and fifty-two minutes.

When have I ever been able to give him so much time in the past?

It's as though I'm attending my own funeral.

My room is filled with the scent of lilies and roses.

After my father had been told about his cancer he became angry when a flower delivery arrived.

'After all, I'm not dead yet!'

I think it's wonderful.

People come to visit me and strange things happen.

One late afternoon my two lives meet on my bed.

Ulrica and Carin are here. Their father has made the trip, accompanied by his daughter from a marriage before his and mine. She, for whom I once sang lullabies – like me, much too young to be a stepmother – wants to show me her newborn baby girl. They have brought with them a bunch of flowers from his current girlfriend. Pontus and Gustaf run in and out. Olle is pottering about in the next room, and the girls are sitting on the edge of the bed.

There is no need for words of reconciliation, for we have never been anything other than friends.

We talk about everyday things. About mutual friends and events of the day.

It feels good.

There is a lot that is not said.

But it isn't needed either.

It lies beneath the surface and I know that it is kind.

On another occasion, Mimmi and I are hostesses for a gentlemen's lunch. Six gentlemen from the newsroom's editorial desk kiss my cheek and hug me as I sit in the armchair with an extra cushion at my back.

We serve an old-fashioned Swedish speciality: fatty sausage, slowly fried over a low heat, stewed potatoes, beer and caraway-flavoured schnapps.

Almost nothing of what I say is audible over the hum of voices, but that doesn't matter. I'm happy and know that my friends from work will come back soon.

One Saturday afternoon my friend the musician arrives, and sings unaccompanied, just for me.

Somewhere over the rainbow way up high,
There's a land that I heard of once in a lullaby.

Then we laugh and cry, indiscriminately.

When we say goodbye we know we shall never see each other again.

'Not in this world,' she says.

The chaplain I met in hospital says that moments of total closeness and total friendship belong to eternity.

'It's a glimpse of eternity at any rate,' she says.

Nowadays Gustaf only wants to talk about the bronze age. The stone age is finished with and the children are practising Christmas songs.

Ulrica arrives from Lund. This is nice, because she hasn't been in contact as often as usual.

'It's because I'm sad. I think about you all the time. Always. But I'm afraid you might have to comfort me.'

'I'll comfort you willingly. We can comfort each other.'

'Yes, but you're worse off than I am.'

'I wouldn't be too sure about that. It's probably much worse for you than for me.'

'But I feel I have to be strong and pull myself together. I'm the eldest child. When people ask me how you are, I always answer rationally, give an account of your condition. And if anyone asks how I feel, I answer in the same way. It's only when I'm on my own that I can be sad. I find it hard to be sad in front of others. Really sad. I have unbelievable control over myself. In front of my friends, I'm only as sad as I think they can take,' says she. My eldest.

It sounds like a description of me before I became ill and let go: in control, disciplined.

I have passed this on to my daughter.

The chaplain spoke about the positive changes that can take place now.

I hope Ulrica will dare to rebel.

Four children and four different ways of reacting.

What does Pontus mean? Is he just being funny? Is he trying to cheer me up? Is he downright angry, feeling left in the lurch by his mother?

'Mummy, let's play rugby later, and some American football. You're good at tackling.'

I start to laugh in the way that people with ALS do: like a braying donkey. It's the bulbar factor.

'Yes, but, Mummy, I can take that tube and hold it, so there won't be any problem when you want to make a tackle!

'Mummy, can you become a newsreader again? "There was an accident today in Åkersberga and two men were killed by a woman".'

'No, I can't.'

'Yes, you can! You can if you have the will. You have to think positively!'

'That's true almost all the time.'

'But, Mummy, another thing, can't we do a trip round the world? You row and I'll eat pizza, like the first people on earth. A fish can be the motor.'

'Why are you talking like this?' I ask, anxiety seeping into me.

'Because I want to do these things with you!'

'But I'm ill!'

'You can if you have the will,' he exclaims.

'I'm not going to give up! You can play the piano. *Für Elise*. Or sing opera. *Carmen*. Mummy, tomorrow we'll pull out that tube and have a party. Stand up and we'll walk to your bed. Keep fighting!'

'I can't.'

'Yes you can. It'll work if you have the will.'

God, give me strength!

'OK, we'll agree on that! See you tomorrow. Night-night.'

A lot of dexterity exists in the head of a paralysed person. A way of remembering. Rather like the starved prisoner who fantasizes about delicacies.

Or acts of love he has experienced.

I make notes.

Some pretty paper and a fountain pen of good quality. My signature. A little curve on *a*. Link together *n* and *l*. The *q* looks stylish, and the *t* is as lighthearted as a major key. Finally the dots over the *i*s.

I wrap up the parcels.

Hear the crackle of the paper as I cut it. Wind string around it. And then the bow. Loop, wind round, loop and pull.

I knit.

Cast on. Knit purl and plain. I'm not very good at it, but it's good practice.

I cook.

Slice garlic, pull off scented thyme leaves and lay them with olive oil and sea salt on a substantial piece of cod.

I polish copper.

I caress.
Drive the car.
Clean mushrooms.
Weed.
Cast a bowline.
Put putty on window-frames.
In my memory.
So I don't forget.

It's as though it's all falling into place now.

My home is totally adapted to my disability with a lift, wheelchairs, carers, ramps, lavatories, a hospital bed and God knows what else.

I have now received a page-turner, which sometimes works. At worst it reduces a page to pulp. I have to give it the signal to turn as soon as I begin a new page: it's that slow.

But it's important that such things are available. Not everyone is as impatient as me.

The centre for disability appliances has given me a computer I control with a little reflector on the tip of my nose, which 'presses down' the key.

It's good.

I just have to learn how to get my thoughts to go through my nose instead of my fingers.

Gustaf is also starting to adapt and understand. This is as it should be, but it stabs and cuts me when he asks, 'Mimmi, will you come home to us even afterwards when Mummy is dead?'

The moon has come a full circle again and casts its silver over the water. I fall asleep in its cold light, and when I wake after 7.5 milligrams of sleeping tablet, the heavens are purple. It is chilly and the mist is rising out of the sea when Pontus finds his mittens at last.

Gustaf's eczema is better and he looks calm when he hears 'yes' in answer to his question.

It tears my heart. I am leaving my sons when they are as little as my daughters were when I was divorced.

'I'm so sad that my children won't have a granny,' says Ulrica, and burrows her head close to mine.

'I am too. I had begun to fantasize about them.'

She leaves for her student lodgings in Lund.

'You won't die when I'm not with you?'

'No, of course not.'

(For surely I will feel it when the time comes?)

We have time to conclude things now. Time to remember.

'Mummy, I remember once when you farted.'

'Me? Never.'

'It's true. I was two and stood behind your gigantic bum.'

'I haven't got a gigantic bum.'

'When I was little it was to me.'

She imitates how it sounded.

'It's my first memory. You had on lilac dungarees.'

'Oh, well, that explains it. I was pregnant.'

Barbara Sterner, the counsellor on the ALS team at the Karolinska Hospital, meets relatives as well as patients, and she knows a lot about how they may react.

The other day she met my Gustaf. They offered each other English sweets and Dime bars, and talked for an hour.

'He's a thinker, your youngest,' she said.

'The lady I met, her sister died and she had a twelve-year-old boy,' Gustaf told me afterwards.

Perhaps I can find out later what else they talked about.

The counsellor knows that the relatives often have a worse time than the patient.

'To watch powerlessly while a loved one slowly gets weaker is awful. To grieve and at the same time to make the most of each day. Of the time one still has. One prepares oneself consciously and unconsciously for the loss one knows will come. In despair one can be anything but sympathetic and tolerant.'

I put questions to her by email and she replies in detail:

Children need to have as normal a life as possible during the parent's illness. A strong network of calm people who are truly there for them is invaluable. Children need normality, and one should be careful about 'stigmatizing' more than is necessary at school etc. This doesn't mean that one should hide things from the child. On the contrary, one must take into account what stage each child is at, as far as his or her development is concerned. Children never completely lose hope that the parent will be miraculously cured. So it is pointless to try to get the child to process the parent's impending death.

Children often show clearly what they are prepared to take in. Don't insist, since they have undeveloped defence mechanisms. This is true, to a great degree, of teenagers as well. They often change the subject when the pressure is too great, and then you should follow the child and not transgress their limits. Showing that you understand how they feel and being open to questions when they arise usually goes a long way.

'How do you feel about your patients?'

I can identify with them without any problem, what has happened to them could at any time happen to me. But suddenly to have to face a terminal illness, which has nothing to do with heredity and which you haven't caused yourself, whether by eating, drinking or smoking – it's almost impossible to imagine.

For each person I meet who has received their diagnosis, I am amazed by how they, each one in his or her own way, succeed in setting up strategies that allow them to live a life full of meaning, in many cases deeper meaning, during the time that is left to them.

I ask myself continually how far my own capacity would stretch if it were put to the test.

'Is this palliative care?' I ask the doctor with the yellow plaits. She is sitting at my bedside and we have time to talk while the morphine is taking effect.

'Yes. It's all about alleviating symptoms. We help people with incurable illnesses. Nobody should have to feel pain.'

'Have you any other ALS patients?'

'No, you're the only one. I read up on your illness before I came here. It isn't very common. We usually have cancer cases.'

My frail little body is put to bed in warmth and down. The pain in my stomach melts away.

The hole with the umbilical cord is giving a little trouble.

In the next room the boys are playing computer games. The smell of Bolognese sauce wafts from the kitchen.

I am at home in my bed. In fact it's not mine, but the county council's. The mattress is made of black rubber balls filled with air. It helps prevent bedsores, which very ill and immobile people can get.

It's been used before.

A week ago I was registered with ACH, Advanced Care at Home. It is almost seven months since I received my diagnosis of amyotrophic lateral sclerosis.

Palliative care to alleviate suffering and improve the quality of life when cure is no longer an option. It is care in the final stage of life.

'The quality of life' – why not 'the quality of death'? The patient is enabled to complete their life with dignity, close to those they love.

I lie amid down and pillows and hear how life goes on in the house. Without me, it will continue.

'Have you finished your homework?'

'Yes, Daddy.'

'Come on, then, supper's ready.'

'What are we having?'

My husband, the father of my sons, has started to cook. Nothing is impossible.

He has got hold of an extra-granny, who helps with homework. It's sensible that she is here while I still am. Here.

If she is in a hurry, the doctor with the yellow plaits doesn't show it. She gives me her time, even though she is freelance.

What is interesting about working with the dying?

My neurologist says, 'Interesting is not the right word, even if I have used it. These are the encounters within the medical sphere that feel important. Encounters with a patient who has an incurable illness, who only has a little time left, are more than interesting. They demand a lot of you, both in knowledge and empathy. These are situations in which you come close to death, as a doctor and as a human being, and they are overwhelming experiences, granted to relatively few.

'To work as a doctor is a privilege, with all the contact it gives, all the insights into life, dying and death. Sometimes you find it extremely moving, at others just very moving.

'It affects me as a human being. Perhaps I can begin to understand what is important in life and what means less.'

I, so deeply involved in how my life is ending, am grateful that these people exist.

To be given someone's time. That someone has time for me.

That is a gift so great, so great.

A colleague comes to our home and reads aloud from a good novel in his beautiful voice.

He sits beside my bed where I am lying while the tube-food is pumped in. We have lit a candle and I don't want the book to end, ever.

Another asks if she can bring along a woman friend.

'She'll be good for you.'

I meet a woman with extensive experience of life. I have read and been fascinated by a couple of her books. Now she is sitting with me and I promise to buy an espresso machine for the next time she comes.

'Everything here is good except the coffee.' She laughs.

There is a tacit understanding that we will talk about spirituality, but she gasps when I ask, 'What is your relationship with God?'

I am embarrassed when I realize that the question was too direct.

'For me it is more intimate than sexuality. I melt and feel fulfilled. My heart becomes as soft as butter.'

She grew up in a Jewish home and has always felt that academic excellence was expected of her.

'But now it is more important to be good than to be clever.'

She speaks about the two paths: that of fear and that of love.

I think that perhaps this is what I was thinking when I decided not to let the disease gnaw my thoughts to pieces and make me bitter. When I decided to live in the present.

We talk about tasting the darkness, seeing it, touching it. Darkness is real, but it is not all there is.

'I can exist in darkness, but I am not my darkness. I am so very much more,' she says. 'I know that something else exists. I can reach a deep acceptance and open myself to the present and to love.'

That is what she says, Anita Goldman – she drinks my coffee anyway – and that is what I think too.

She is writing a book about Etty, a woman who was murdered in Auschwitz. Etty writes in her diary:

To suffer is not beneath human dignity. I mean that one can suffer with human dignity and without human dignity. I mean that most Westerners do not understand the art of suffering and are instead gripped by a thousand different kinds of anguish . . . One must accept that death is a part

*of life, even the most terrible death. And do we not live a
whole life every day, and does it then make any great difference if we live a few days more or less?*

When Anita leaves, she turns in the doorway. 'We are
all going to walk the same road as you. Make the same
journey. You are doing it now with an open mind. You
will encounter a bright future.'

Another of my friends knows a child psychiatrist. He
comes to my home, drinks the coffee without a murmur,
and likes the ginger biscuits.

He is very tall and very grey, and he touches on what
is important for me.

'It is essential that you are part of your children's lives,
and that you tell them what you need and want for them
and from them. They ought to keep your expectations in
mind.

'Settle your grievances, if there are any.'

And about children's grief: 'They often move from
space to space. The everyday space. The space for sorrow.
We adults let grief entwine with all other feelings. For
children it's different, and that may seem odd to us, since
we have different feelings in the same space.'

Roses, of course, are always roses, but best of all is that
someone gives their time. That someone shares their
knowledge with me.

A good conversation.

One day a friend arrives and offers me her hands. The room is fragrant with aromatic oils. It is so pleasurable that I fall asleep on the massage table that she has dragged all the way up the narrow staircase.

It is too strange. The truth is that I would not wish to be without this part of my life!

The time I have left here is extremely limited.

But it is now for the first time that I feel myself to be living in the present.

Death brings me closer to life.

On the net, I carry on a conversation about life with my younger daughter, Carin. She is now twenty-one and it was ages ago when I, just having delivered her, wondered how I would make a pair of trousers with space for the tumour. Since then we have survived teenage rebellion and a lot more besides. But she must tell that story herself.

These are extracts from one of her letters.

You asked me what we talked about last Friday evening. You asked me what I am learning from this and what it is that makes me strong. This letter is about precisely that. Because these are questions that are not at all easy to answer off the cuff.

You were a bird that flew from twig to twig, seeking something else, something new. Too full of anxiety to stop. Perhaps it was a search for confirmation. Confirmation that you were good enough, confirmation that you were loved, confirmation that you were really alive.

A search for love. A search for yourself. You were like the flame of a giant, long-life candle, so bright and blazing, so full of energy.

But you were tired. I saw and felt that you were tired. You had to be as everyone wanted you to be, to be adequate. You made no demands, because you were a good girl and good girls do not make demands . . . You tried to keep everything together. Small boys, work and teenage rebellion. You believed that you had superpowers, but you didn't have superpowers because you were a dove, a frail dove of peace.

Out of the dove, an eagle was born.

The eagle is powerful, proud and protective. It lifts its wings and carries itself over the land, the world, the oceans, some stormy, others calm. The wings will carry you all the way into eternity.

The eagle that was born of a dove grew out of a feeling of freedom from danger that is present in the illness. You know now what you have got, and you feel our love for you. You are starting to find yourself . . . because you can't hide yourself any longer, and you don't want to hide yourself any longer . . . You have become so strong and full of the joys of life . . . You are more alive than many other people. Because you make the most of your time and live every second of your life filled with love. A mental awareness. In your dying you teach me how to live . . . There is an eagle in every soul . . .

You teach us how frail life is.

You teach us to stop for a while and talk, to hear and see each other.

You teach us to love.

You teach us to use our sense of humour.

You teach us about loss, grief, fear and death.

You teach us to live and why we are alive.

A question to you: what is death?

Un abrazo
Carin

The vicar whose son builds churches with his toy bricks gives me a prayer cloth that smells of herbs.

She sings about not being afraid, and we remember how we pushed our prams uphill in the winter slush.

'You should feel angry. You have the right to complain,' she says, and quotes the hymn-book version of Martin Luther: ' "You must learn to cry out, and not just sit there on your own or lie on a bench, hanging your head and letting your thoughts chew and gnaw at you . . ." '

She is the one who will scatter earth over me, and when I think about that I am carried away to a chapel near a white beach where towering waves roll in from the Norwegian sea.

In that sand there are no tracks.

We get there by crossing a precipitously deep fjord in a little fishing-boat from Reine in southernmost Lofoten.

On the vertical cliffs, at the foot of Helvetistinden, the three-toed gull nests, and lots of puffins with their comical red-and-white beaks cross our path.

The girls complain over the steep, stony path that takes

us from the village of Vindstad towards the open sea to the west. They are still small and it is a couple of years before the boys arrive.

Up on the summit there is a little graveyard with simple crosses and an old woman with a rake.

Her face has been battered by the winds and her gaze, turned to the horizon, is steely grey when she tells of the storm that took her husband and a few other men. She lets the rake touch the gravel. Unnecessary words are seldom uttered up here. That winter was severe and not even the Gulf Stream could keep the cold at bay.

'He had to lie here in the shed until the thaw had come and we could bury him in the earth.'

My vicar, now at my sickbed, says she understands my longing for the sea.

Olle does too, but he wants a place to go to with the children, to remember and lay some flowers.

That makes me happy.

However.

Which place on earth is my home?

Where do I feel at home?

The vicar says that her children have asked if she wants to be buried whole or burnt to ashes.

'Dear me, what on earth did you reply?'

'Buried whole.'

Her experience is that that is easier for children to understand.

'Mummy is lying there in the coffin and they can do drawings to put in. It will be a lovely moment and I can sing and play the guitar.'

I remember then when my granny died after a year in a geriatric ward. We were to say farewell beside the coffin and her jaw had fallen open. This dignified, stately woman gaped, and I recoiled, scared.

But that was then, with an undertaker in black, watching the clock.

I think about the hare and the bird we buried at our country house the previous summer, how it was completely natural and there was nothing remarkable about their decomposing.

It is probably possible to become reconciled to that.

'And it becomes just a parting. A ceremony. It is real for the children,' says the vicar.

Just north of Lofoten lies Troms county. In a village on the way to the North Cape, Olle has a job as a doctor, for the month of July. There are no really old houses there. This is not because the sea has ravaged their wooden frames, but because the Germans burnt down the village during the war.

One house is supposed to have been spared since the man who lived there said that they would have to set him on fire too.

Late one evening, we are eating cod baked in the oven with olive oil, tarragon and lemon, when the telephone rings.

'Can the doctor come? My brother isn't very well.'

The bag is packed and nothing is very far away in the village.

There is one room and a kitchen, and two men aged about sixty-five.

One is lying still on the floor, and although Olle injects adrenaline straight into his heart, no life returns.

'Your brother is dead,' says Olle, and I find the instant coffee in the kitchen.

It is not advisable to move somebody who is lying dead at home on the floor in case the police want to investigate. All three of us have to step over the dead brother while the water boils and telephone calls are made.

'You can bury him,' say the emergency services, far away. They have neither the time nor the energy to suspect a crime.

When we try today to remember what make of car the undertaker had, we believe it was a large old American one.

It was black, with a cross on the roof and curtains with frills at the windows.

'I'm the summer locum.'

'So am I,' Olle greets her.

She is so small, so young and thin, and she seems to have borrowed the regular undertaker's suit.

Olle is writing the death certificate and is fully occupied with that.

She is lost and turns to me.

'Can you help me?'

'Of course.'

She, so tiny, and I lift the man on to the stretcher, with dignity and care, and we carry him out to the car.

It is after midnight above the Arctic Circle. The sun is shining brightly, close to the moon, when the hearse glides down the side of the mountain.

That is something I think about quite often. How close to death one is in the wilds of the countryside and at sea. I am drawn to memories of mortality.

'How do you feel about God?' wonders my so constant friend Birgit. She travels three hundred and fifty kilometres to visit me every month.

I have no answer.

My grandmother's generation forbids me to question the idea. It feels punishable not to believe.

'I feel safe,' I reply, and have to spell out the word 'safe' since my tongue is as it is.

'Perhaps it's the same thing,' she suggests cautiously.

'Perhaps it is a premonition of something.'

She and Ulrica sit close to me, and we talk about the funeral. Birgit tells us about a father who died and how the children and his wife decorated the coffin with lichen, moss and stones that he had walked on over the years.

I like the idea. It would also be good for the children.

We exchange thoughts about grief. About how one can be at different levels of grief in a family. If one person seems especially sad, someone else has to hold back their own sorrow for a while. It often works like this unconsciously, without one thinking about it.

'Everyone can't cry at the same time. When you're sad I have to pull myself together and be strong,' as Olle often says.

But sometimes I want to protest.

'Your grief can also be my comfort.'

Shared weeping can soothe.

I grieve a lot now. Alone.

Will the sum of my life be this illness?

Will the images of me as a healthy mother, woman, wife and friend crumble away?

Will Gustaf, the youngest, ever remember a living mummy?

Will sorrow stand in the way of everything that has been good?

It is when melancholy wants to root itself in the December darkness, when the smell of mulled wine wafts up to me, in bed with my nutrition tube, that I feel bitterness creeping up.

It is at this point that Mimmi happens to scratch my hand.

'Ow!'

My weak left hand suddenly acquires the strength to lash out at hers.

I hit my friend.

And no apology springs to my lips.

What is happening?

A little scratch upsets me.

The powerlessness of being unable to make myself understood is limitless.

I hide myself behind bulletproof glass and feel no sense of safety.

The palliative home-nursing team, who alleviate all kinds of pain, know that it is good for the patient to talk to an outsider.

I receive a visit from a conversational therapist.

'I recognize your anger so well from other sick people. It is such a disappointment to be crippled as you are. Many people, even those who can speak, react like that. But it is hard for those who are close to you. And to be cared for by a friend can be tricky. Are you seriously angry with her?'

'No,' I reply, and start to sob.

'Why are you upset?'

It tears me apart and wears me down, but in the end I manage to say it.

'Because Pontus asked her, not me, for sticking-plaster and sympathy when he hurt himself.'

'You feel that others are taking over?'

'Yes.'

This was clearly a reaction that welled up in the

reptilian part of my brain. Not worth analysing, really. But normal for someone who has lost her grip on something she is used to holding on to.

Accordingly, I forgive myself.

'What is happening in your life now?' wonders my friend with the white hair. He gazes at me intensely with his beautiful dark brown eyes.

I look away and my eye is caught by the neighbours' strings of Christmas lights. I could talk about the strangers who lift me on to the lavatory during the night, about the food that upsets my stomach, about the phlegm in my throat that I have ever greater difficulty in coughing up and about how troublesome and laborious speaking has become.

Inside myself I see instead an open door.

'Am on my way into a new room.'

'What can you see?'

'Two pillars, one solemnity and the other solitude. I am alone in the room, and there is yet another door. I do not feel afraid or abandoned, but full of sorrow.'

The conversational therapist said the other day that grief often feels lonely. Part of the work of grieving has to be done by oneself. Nobody can be of any help with the innermost sorrow. One must bear it on one's own.

He listens and nods, and he is about to talk to me about when his father died, when the door bursts open and Gustaf storms in. He stops abruptly and stares, amazed.

'Mummy! You look just like an ordinary person!'

I am sitting in a leather armchair that the hospital has sent. It was bought by a man who had ALS; in his will he donated it to others with the same diagnosis.

'In that chair you look like my usual old mum. Cool!'

What a saving grace my sons and daughters are. What life-extenders.

With them, I am not alone.

Gustaf takes a bite of his biscuit, then calls to the extra-granny, and my friend with the white hair begins to talk about his father.

'I held his hand, and his eye – he only had one – stared hard at me. We sat like that and stared fixedly at each other. I stared at his eye and he stared at me. We built a bridge between our eyes. It was so powerful it was almost tangible. After a while, his eye formed a tunnel. I followed him into his being, his inner self, and it was a peculiar feeling.

'And then he died.

'The tunnel was no longer there.

'I was filled with a sensation that he had overflowed into me.'

'What an experience.'

'When my mother died it was quite different. It was a

warm day in August. We sat beside her bed. She died after a long struggle, with the window wide open. Suddenly a rush of wind swept in. *Hyyueee, hyyueee.*

'And afterwards it was utterly silent.

'It was as though she had puffed the wind out of her body,' he ended.

After this we sit silently for a while, and what he has said sinks in. I hear our extra-granny get going on Pontus's maths problems. Gustaf, who has finished, rushes up the stairs and jerks open the door again.

'Mummy, are you coming to school for the St Lucia ceremony?'

'No, I can't. Daddy and Ulrica are going with you instead.'

'Oh, good! I'd only be teased if you came. Nobody else in my class has their mummy in a wheelchair.'

'Oh, really!'

'Yes. It's OK, Mummy. It's good and bad. Bad that you're sick, I mean.'

'OK.'

I let it go, don't reproach him. Don't want to make him feel guilty. We can talk later about how anyone could end up in a wheelchair.

And I understand him.

You get symptoms that indicate illness. You swing to and fro between hope and despair. It might, of course, be a mistake. Perhaps I'm imagining it all.

But the insight is real enough. A person knows when she is sick. When Death is trying on his suit.

It has been over two years since the spoon wobbled because my hand trembled when I drank Thai soup at a restaurant on the Boulevard St Laurent in Montréal.

I thought at the time, a person knows when she is sick. Death snaps at my heels.

Thank goodness hope took over: it's only a nerve under pressure.

Time passes, the symptoms get worse and so does the chaos that ensues. Then the diagnosis is made. I am terminally ill. Certainty and confirmation.

Those around me get used to the idea. Everyone, wherever they are, establishes mile-stones towards the end.

I have already passed one of mine.

Everyone around me accepts that their mother/wife/ friend is bedridden.

And perhaps soon nobody will remember her as healthy.

I am so afraid of that.

Gustaf, do you remember that you rode on my shoulders when we ran down all – all – the stairs of the Eiffel Tower? You were five years old and my back was so strong. It was the day before Pontus lost his toy squirrel, Korre, in the pool under the world-famous bridge in Claude Monet's garden at Giverny. I pulled off my trousers and jumped in among the waterlilies and got a scolding from a guard. In schoolgirl French I explained our dilemma. The guard rolled up his uniform trousers and became a hero when he handed over a wet cloth squirrel to Pontus.

You who are still young, do you remember your healthy mummy?

Perhaps I ought not to indulge in memories. Last night I dreamt about white envelopes, large and of good quality. I bought them from Eivor in the bookshop. Blank white sheets of paper and envelopes of the best kind. It can only mean that I must put my affairs in order. Clearly.

So dreary. I'll do it later.

People react so differently to serious illness. Someone who visited me or rang daily six months ago doesn't come any more. He gets depressed at the sight of me. Others, however, come in from the sidelines and give of themselves.

More come than stay away.

Relationships are sorely tried when someone, particularly a woman, becomes ill. I heard about a man, someone in this area, who separated from his wife when she was seriously ill with cancer. It was so tough for him to see her in such a state after thirty years of marriage, people said.

If a couple hasn't felt intimate, genuine closeness beforehand it can be tricky. The one who is sick often feels guilty, the one who stands by her side, inadequate.

At that point it is easy to give up and flee fear.

I know of a woman who longed to make a garland with her husband. Everyone knew she would die before the spring. She wanted to get close to him and share memories with him, everything that had existed between them.

She wanted to weave a garland of beautiful scented blossoms and sharp, bitter herbs. Some of these plants had not yet been picked, and it was time to harvest them.

She wanted to sort every stem and find sweetness even in the most bitter ones.

But he couldn't cope. Perhaps he didn't want to. Or was he afraid?

Yes, well, I don't know how it ended. All that is certain is that you can't make that sort of garland alone.

Dawn, on the day before Christmas Eve 2003, fills me with wonder. The condensation between the window-panes has frozen and through the ice-blossoms I can see the sea steaming in the coldness of the air.

It is so astonishingly beautiful.

The sky is flushed purple and pink. One or two stars are still twinkling palely. When the sun rises above the forest of firs, a rainbow appears and the gulls seem whiter than usual.

I am back at home after four days in a hospice, a nursing-home for the care of the dying. The average length of stay is twenty days. Half of the patients die there.

'The room with the bier – can I see it?' I ask, when rest-lessness takes root in me.

Surprised, the nurse pushes me to a room with a bur-bling fountain. The walls are yellow, and at one of the narrow ends clouds have been painted in earthy colours. In the corner sits an angel. The floor is paved with terra-cotta tiles. I am convinced that there is a drainage culvert under that object, which reminds me of the cradle that my brother, I and all our children have lain in.

Although this one is much longer. And has no bottom.

It is lined with dark, rust-red fabric, which reaches to the stone floor. I start to think about my grandfather and when I ate raspberry bonbons with him instead of going to my piano lessons with Anna Palmér, in Kristinehamn.

I can't play the piano now either.

When the image of my dead grandfather has faded, I snivel: 'Why?'

'You're wondering why it's so narrow. It's not a bed. It's for a stretcher.'

There are three doors into the room. We came in through one, the second goes to a mortuary and the third to a separate driveway outside.

I have difficulty in calming my sobbing. There is so much, there are so many, in this room. And the bier frightens me.

But I am glad to have seen it, the room with the bier.

The nursing-home is very nice, although it makes me feel gravely ill. That I am gravely ill has been a fact for a long time. Still, I can forget it for short periods when I am at home.

Christmas is here, and a year ago when I got into a tangle and fumbled with the parcels, the spectre said that was my last Christmas.

It was wrong.

My daughters and sons are close by me. We know that this is for real now. Having them here, skin to skin, makes my joy so strong that I don't need to pretend to be merry.

My four children, my husband, my mother-in-law, Mimmi, her son Hugo and I celebrate Christmas together. The table is extravagantly laden with pickled herring, ham, oven-baked potato-and-anchovy gratin, salmon, brown cabbage, red cabbage, green cabbage, swede, sausages, meatballs, boiled dried fish, pancakes with saffron, and of course ham-broth dip, which only my mother-in-law likes. I can smell the scents of caraway, dried Seville orange peel and wormwood.

'I can't understand how you can sit with us at the table when you can't taste a single crumb,' says Mimmi.

It might seem strange, but it doesn't bother me. I can taste the smells and remember my childhood's special-occasion meatballs, prepared from minced veal and sour cream by my granny's cook. I remember the Christmas ham, which was laid in a solution of salt, sugar, saltpetre, Spanish pepper, ginger, bay leaves, red onions and allspice as early as the first Sunday in Advent, ready to be boiled on 'the day before ham-broth dipping day', Christmas Eve. It lasted until after Twelfth Night, and when it began to go off, it was baked again and considered as good as new.

That was then. Now we tie a red satin ribbon round my sterile nutrient solution hanging from the drip frame, decorated with Christmas glitter and garlands made of plastic balls.

I haven't eaten any proper food for two months, haven't even drunk anything. The tiniest sip of water goes down the wrong way. I have problems swallowing my own saliva, and almost every evening the district nurses come to give me a morphine injection, which dries the phlegm and stops me coughing.

One day the lady vicar arrives, she who is to scatter earth. She comes with a lantern and a Christmas tree with gingerbread angels she has baked. When we turn our backs, Mimmi's labrador eats them. All except one.

'My Rufs would have done that too,' says the vicar, comfortingly. She reads the Christmas gospel at my bedside.

Many people come on a Christmas visit. It's fun, but they behave differently. I can't speak at all now, so they raise their voices and articulate their words extra-clearly. I have lost some of my facial mobility, so I am sometimes met by blank gazes. If I speak, even though I shouldn't, I have to make such an effort that I seem angry.

'Why are you yelling like that?'

Nowadays I receive pats on the cheek or, worst of all, on the head, like a child. I hate that condescending pity. So distant from sympathy and empathy.

At Christmas one may make a wish, and I know what I can't get enough of: closeness, warmth, truth and trust.

I want so much to remember things, events, together. Don't pity me. Whisper secrets in my ear. Your secrets. Ours.

I'm serious.

Don't flee from me. Don't be afraid.

It's not that bad.

It's only me, you know.

The smell of tar lingers in the woodwork of the jetty, and from the beach I can sniff reeds and mouldering leaves.

The water is cold and I want to believe that the last vestiges of ice are starting to melt.

When I was very little, and the winters were harsh, my father and the other men used to saw metre-thick blocks from the ice on Lake Vänern. They carted them with ropes and pulleys to the forest of firs, to a place the sun never reached. The patterns, bubbles and lace in the deep-frozen water were the most beautiful things I had ever seen. I felt loss when the blocks were lowered into the sawdust in the little cold storage bunker with the ladder up to the opening in the roof. In this ice-tomb, milk, cheese and sauna-smoked ham were kept fresh during the summer holidays.

With a sense of wonder, I walk out now on to the jetty of my memories and hope I will feel at peace all the way out.

Water gave me birth. The sea is my source of primordial power.

It sustains me.

The sea will sustain you too, Ulrica, Carin, Pontus and Gustaf.

A fresh wind is blowing from the shore when I untie the half-hitch and put out to sea.

The sea is choppy, with little white horses.

I settle myself comfortably on the deck and wait.

The wind rows me out, and I am at peace.

When it slackens at dusk I will have reached my haven.

Every second is a life.

Ulla-Carin Lindquist died peacefully at her home
on 10 March 2004